POWER YOGA
for BEGINNERS

LIZ LARK

author of *Yoga for Beginners*

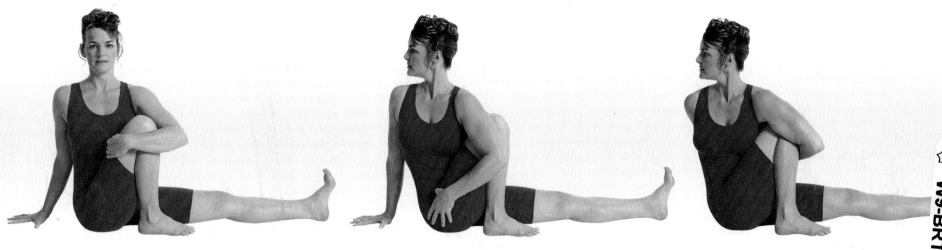

HarperResource
An Imprint of HarperCollinsPublishers

CREATED AND PRODUCED BY:
Carroll & Brown Limited
20 Lonsdale Road
London NW6 6RD

FIRST PUBLISHED IN THE USA IN 2003 BY:
HarperResource, an imprint of HarperCollins Publishers

EDITOR: Kelly Thompson
DESIGNER: Justin Ford
EDITORIAL ASSISTANTS: Stuart Moorhouse, Tom Broder
PRODUCTION STAFF: Karol Davies, Nigel Reed, Paul Stradling

PHOTOGRAPHER: Jules Selmes
PHOTOGRAPHIC ASSISTANT: David Yems

POWER YOGA FOR BEGINNERS
Text copyright © 2003 Liz Lark
Compilation Copyright © 2003 Carroll & Brown Ltd, London

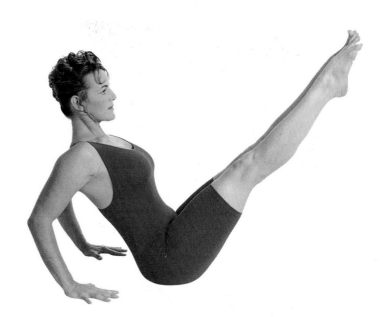

For information address HarperCollins Publishers, Inc.
10 East 53rd Street, New York, NY 10022.

HarperCollins books may be purchased for educational, business, or sales promotional use. For information, please write: Special Markets Department, HarperCollins Publishers, Inc. 10 East 53rd Street, New York, NY 10022.

FIRST EDITION
Library of Congress Cataloging-in-Publication Data is available upon request

ISBN 0-06-053541-5

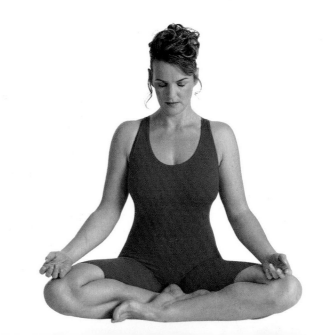

The exercises in this book are safe if performed as described, but you should consult your doctor before beginning this or any other exercise program, especially if you have an existing medical condition. Neither the exercises nor the information given with them are intended to replace medical advice. If you have any concerns about your health, consult your doctor. Neither the author nor the publishers shall be liable or responsible for any loss, injury, or damage allegedly arising from any information or suggestion in this book.

Contents

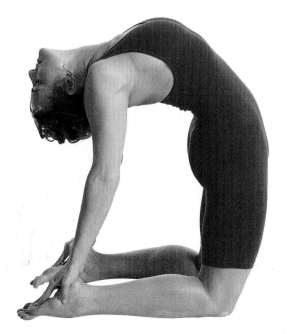

Introduction

Yoga is becoming increasingly popular all over the world as a means of developing a stronger, leaner body. Improving personal appearance is a positive by-product of practice, but yoga, meaning "to unite" is also an ideal way to become more balanced and relaxed in today's fast-moving society. It not only strengthens and enhances your physical body and health, but also allows you to discover your full potential on a psychological and spiritual level.

You don't need any previous experience to follow this foundation program of power yoga postures at home. But read the introduction before beginning your practice, and do the postures in the order given.

THE BENEFITS OF YOGA

If practiced regularly with patience and awareness, yoga can:

- Realign your body on a skeletal level
- Improve your posture
- Strengthen your bones
- Cleanse and tone your muscles
- Stimulate better blood circulation
- Help remove toxins from your body
- Provide a deep massage, improving internal bodily functions, including digestion and respiration
- Enhance emotional well-being
- Increase confidence and self-esteem
- Soothe your mind and decrease anxiety

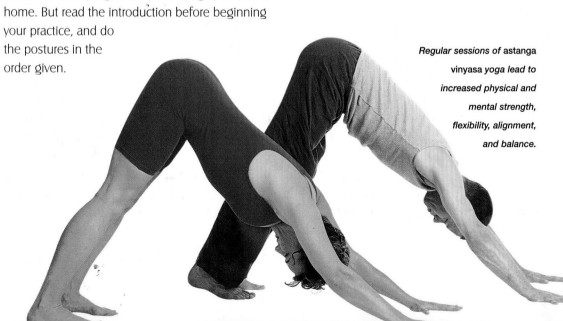

Regular sessions of astanga vinyasa *yoga lead to increased physical and mental strength, flexibility, alignment, and balance.*

HOW YOGA WORKS

The age-old, Eastern movements involved in yoga postures intensely work and stretch your muscles, and exercise your joints. They also awaken the latent energy (*kundalini*) that lies at the bottom of your spine, transforming it into a rejuvenating life-force (*prana*) flowing throughout your body, and creating or renewing a sense of well-being within you. This cleansing of your energy channels (*nadis*) not only causes your body to soften and open, but also has the same effect on your mind, leaving you with an increased sense of calm and clarity. So following the yoga program in this book will help you cultivate an awareness of your own mind and body, and develop a deep sense of internal steadiness.

What is Power Yoga?

Power Yoga—a modern term for traditional *astanga vinyasa* yoga—is a specific, dynamic branch of classical *hatha* yoga that taps into and circulates vital energy throughout your body. *Astanga* literally means "eight limbs," while *vinyasa* means "breath-connected movement." Thus, *astanga vinyasa* yoga involves doing breath-connected movement to develop certain yogic "limbs" or abilities.

These eight yogic limbs are abstinence, observance, postures (*asana*), breath control (*pranayama*), sense withdrawal (*pratyahara*), concentration, meditation, and absorption. This book is designed to help you cultivate these qualities, concentrating mainly on the key postures and the breath control required to do them.

Astanga vinyasa yoga differs from other forms of yoga in its emphasis on energy seals (*bandhas*). Pages 10–11 will explain these in more detail. These *bandhas* help you achieve deeper breathing, which you should use as the rhythm for your movement. Instead of practicing postures individually and holding each one for a duration, power yoga concentrates just as much on moving smoothly between postures as on the nature of the postures in their own right. This movement on the rhythm of the breath is what links the ordered postures into a dynamic, flowing tapestry that has the power to cleanse, hone, and realign both your mind and body.

THE PARADOX OF POWER IN YOGA

The term "power" in the title may, at first glance, imply achievement, advancement of personal status, or great physical strength. "Power" in the context of yoga actually refers to the internal strength and courage that can be developed through regular, attentive yoga practice.

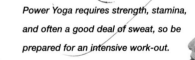

Power Yoga requires strength, stamina, and often a good deal of sweat, so be prepared for an intensive work-out.

HOW TO USE THIS BOOK

This book has been designed with a folding base so that you can prop it up next to you while you work through your yoga program.

Take time to read the introduction thoroughly before starting the postures. It gives you the information you need to carry out the poses safely and effectively to gain the most benefit. Always start with Sun Salutations to warm up your body.

If you don't have time to perform the entire program, which takes approximately one and a half hours, choose one of the shorter programs on page 13. Then open the book at the relevant page and begin.

Each page is dedicated to one posture or sequence of postures. The top page provides background information, including benefits, relevant cautions, important teaching points, and guidance on either your breathing, your gaze, or visualizations. The bottom page breaks down the poses into easy-to-follow steps.

Selection of Postures

The sequence of the postures in this book is based on the traditional *astanga vinyasa* method, as taught by master teacher Sri K. Pattabhi Jois in Mysore, India. It is a well-rounded and safe yet challenging sequence. Practice the poses in the specified order, or, if time is limited, choose a timed session from page 13, so that you still perform a safe and balanced yoga program.

The mainly primary-series sequence to be found in this book includes a full range of standing postures, and a combination of effective balancing, warrior, seated, and finishing poses. These are supplemented with two elegant, second-series backbends, The Locust and The Camel (see pages 70–73), in the seated postures chapter. These not only serve as counterpostures to the primary-series Forward Bends, but also open your chest, and lengthen your spine. Two postures from the advanced series are also included, Lord of the Dance (see pages 50–51) and Warrior 3 (see pages 60–61). And two extra postures—Half-moon (see pages 40–41) and The Eagle (see pages 54–55)—are included to develop your balance. Finally, two valuable relaxation practices are provided.

WHY THESE POSTURES?

Each of the "series" of postures in traditional *astanga vinyasa* yoga has a specific purpose in mind: the primary series is designed to strengthen, align, and empower your body and mind; the more feminine and swan-like second series is designed to cleanse your subtle nervous system; and the advanced series is intended to integrate the immense strength and grace of yoga. Traditionally, second-series postures are not carried out until you have practiced primary series for approximately three years, and advanced postures are only introduced after several years of dedicated practice. However, two poses from advanced series have been included in order to offer a fully integrated, effective foundation practice. But always practice at your own pace: do the Confidence Builders for the more challenging postures if necessary, or leave out these poses to start with, as you will not benefit from a pose if you are straining yourself to do it.

Even when doing challenging postures like Warrior 1, strive to practice with "effortless effort."

EFFORTLESS EFFORT

It is important to practice your postures mindfully, without forcing them or putting any pressure on yourself to achieve certain self-imposed goals. This is because excessive ambition or aggression stimulates your sympathetic nervous system, leading to an overly alert, aroused state. This would be the antithesis of your aim in yoga, which should be to practice calmly, surrendering yourself to your parasympathetic nervous system. So strive to practice with what is called "effortless effort"—a delicate balance between activity and relaxation.

Key Postures

Some postures are referred to frequently throughout this book. Six of these, plus one brief warm-up, are outlined below so that you can make yourself familiar with the basic poses before starting your chosen program.

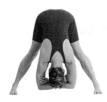

LIGHTNING PREPARATION

Before you begin the Sun Salutations, it is a good idea to do one brief warm-up exercise to prepare your mind and body. Place your feet apart, bend your knees slightly, fold your arms lightly, and bend forward. Hang there for 10–20 breaths, and relax your whole upper body to let the blood flow to your brain.

KEEP YOUR SPINE STRONG

In the Orient, the bamboo embodies fundamental values: strength, simplicity, and purity. The spine, in yogic terms, can be compared to a bamboo: upright and alert, full of energy and vitality, and firm and stable, yet still very flexible. Try throughout your yoga practice to keep your spine as strong, straight, and supple as possible, just like a sanguine bamboo stem.

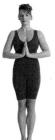

MOUNTAIN (*Tadasana*)

Stand in Mountain by placing your feet together, with your big toes, inner ankles, and inner heels touching. Press your feet firmly into the ground, lift the arches of your feet, tuck your tailbone under, open your chest, draw your lower belly inward, and lift the top of your head skyward. Then bring your arms to the *namaste* gesture (see right).

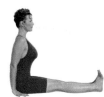

SEATED STAFF (*Dandasana*)

Sit up tall on the floor with your legs stretched out in front of you and with equal weight through both your buttocks. Press the backs of your knees toward the floor, flex your feet, and lift the top of your head skyward.

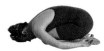

THE CHILD (*Balasana*)

Kneel on the floor, with your buttocks resting on your heels. Then bend your head forward to rest on the floor, with your arms relaxing on the floor beside you, palms turned up.

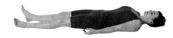

SUPINE (*Savasana*)

Lie down on your back on the floor, and relax both sides of your body. Allow your arms and legs to rest, with your palms facing upward and your toes falling outward. Then close your eyes, relax your jaw, and let your shoulders become heavy.

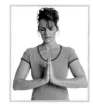

NAMASTE

Place the palms of your hands together at chest-height, so that your lower arms are horizontal and your hands are vertical. Press your hands firmly together. This hand position is also known as the universal peace *mudra*. It helps direct attention to your heartspace, in turn cultivating *bodhicitta*, positive emotional energy.

REVERSE *NAMASTE*

This is the same hand position as above but practiced behind your back. Reach your pinky fingers to touch your back, get your lower arms horizontal, and then press as much of your hands together as possible.

Tools for Power Yoga 1

There are certain aspects specific and integral to *astanga vinyasa* yoga that you should understand before starting the sequence of postures in this book. These will help you gain maximum benefit from each of the postures and deepen your practice over time:

VINYASA

There is a Greek saying that observes: "everything is in flux." This is also true of a deep *astanga vinyasa* practice, as you should flow as smoothly as possible in and out of each pose on your breath, as dictated by the very word *vinyasa*, which means "breath-connected movement." This is why Flow In and Flow Out pictures are provided on each exercise page, and is also why you are guided in your inhalation and exhalation in relation to each movement. Aiming for this continual flux encourages an acceptance within you that nothing in life is fixed, and that everything is mutable. The postures themselves then become living and changing, keeping your mind active and alert.

DRISHTI

The direction of your gaze is known in yoga as *drishti*. Your *drishti* should be directed to one still point in each posture. Focusing on one still point is known as *ekagra*, which helps integrate the left (logical) and the right (intuitive) hemispheres of your brain.

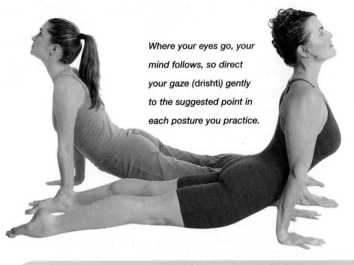

Where your eyes go, your mind follows, so direct your gaze (drishti) gently to the suggested point in each posture you practice.

Apply the concept of "energetic lightness" to the controlled jumps in astanga vinyasa *yoga, such as in the jump-through from Downward Dog to Forward Bend. You should feel as if a harness is pulling your hips skyward, while your hands are firmly rooted to the ground.*

ENERGETIC LIGHTNESS

The term "energetic lightness" refers to a feeling of duality that you should strive for in your practice: of deep grounding through the lower parts of your body, coupled with great transcendence through the upper parts. Avicenna, a thirteenth-century alchemist, used a beautiful metaphor to describe this sensation: an eagle soaring high in the sky had a chain attached to its talons at one end and to a toad on the ground at the other end. This powerful image carried the phrase: "Connect the earthly toad with the heavenly eagle and thou shalt understand the secret of our art." Similarly, constantly striving for "energetic lightness" will help you understand and practice yoga on a deeper level.

UJJAYI BREATHING

The Sanskrit term *ujjayi* means "to stretch the inner breath" or "victorious breathing." This is the breathing technique (*pranayama*) used in *astanga vinyasa* yoga to channel and control your breath in order to calm your mind. Said to increase the absorption of vital energy (*prana*), it involves narrowing the gateway at the back of your throat in order to filter, warm, and refine your breath. Your chest is then filled with this warmed, filtered breath, which expands into the sides of your rib cage, while your lower abdomen is made steady with *uddiyana bandha* (see page 10).

The Nourishing Breath

Developmental psychologist Judith Harris views breathing as the intelligence of the human body: a means to free your body of both emotional and physical tensions. As the breath is such vital food for the mind and body, and as constant awareness of its ebb and flow deepens your ability to be fully present in the moment, it is important to practice it throughout your yoga program, other than during the two relaxation practices at the end.

Ujjayi practice

Take a few moments to practice your *ujjayi* breathing before each yoga practice, until you get used to the feeling it creates. Contract your throat muscles as if you are about to sneeze (*jalandhara bandha*, see page 11), but keep your mouth gently closed. Then breathe in and out through your nose, as smoothly and deeply as you can. The combination of your mouth being closed and the gateway in your throat being contracted may create a soft, sibilant sound, like that of a scuba diver breathing underwater. Do not be surprised or embarrassed by this. It echoes the soothing sound made by ocean waves. Do not worry if you cannot sense the *ujjayi* breath at first. Regular practice with attention to all the key points will soon allow you to progress. Place your hands gently on your abdomen or on your rib cage as you breathe in and out to feel the natural movement that takes place in your body as you do so (see pictures, below and left).

By placing your hands on your rib cage, you can feel it move upward and outward when you inhale, and down and in again when you exhale.

You can either sit cross-legged or lie down on your back to practice your ujjayi breathing—whatever is more comfortable for you.

Tools for Power Yoga 2

BANDHAS

Bandhas are subtle, muscular seals in the body. Although the Sanskrit term *bandha* actually means "lock," their application involves the contraction of certain external muscles in order to "unlock" and contain vital energy within you.

There are many *bandhas*, but in *astanga vinyasa* yoga we are concerned with three—*uddiyana*, *jalandhara*, and *mula*, which are situated in the abdomen, throat, and pelvic area respectively. When harnessed, they activate the latent energy (*kundalini*) at the root of your spine and encourage the flow of vital energy (*prana*) throughout your body. This develops internal awareness and leads to deep relaxation. These seals are an integral part of *astanga vinyasa* yoga practice: they allow you to channel your energy into your breathing and your postures, rather than expending it needlessly.

Learn the *asanas* and the *bandhas* separately at first. Practice them regularly, and only when you feel confident adopting the postures should you try to combine them with your *bandha* practice. It takes a long time to gain a true sense of the *bandhas* at work, so don't worry if you do not feel it at first. The most important thing is that you are aware of them and are gently striving toward them from the start of your practice.

Uddiyana Bandha: abdominal lock

This subtle, internal seal removes sluggishness from your intestines, offers you a fantastic internal massage, and energizes your abdomen and chest. It is also associated with *ujjayi* breathing, because the action of sealing the abdominal wall creates a compression chamber where your upper body can expand, stretch, and channel your breath.

Uddiyana practice

Stand with your feet hip-width apart, your knees bent, your arms pressing onto the tops of your thighs, and your spine straight (see right). Breathe normally to start. Then, after a deep inhalation, exhale deeply, expelling your breath out of your mouth to empty your lungs. Lean over as you do so, tucking your chin toward your chest. Do not inhale, but maintain the exhalation, and draw in your abdomen toward your spine, as if you are wearing an invisible belt that is being pulled more tightly. It should feel like a subtle vacuuming suction. Hold this position for a few seconds without breathing (see far right). Then release, and inhale deeply. It takes regular practice to master this. Repeat it five times, but stop if you feel strained at any time. Do not practice this if you are pregnant, menstruating, or if you have an internally fitted contraceptive device.

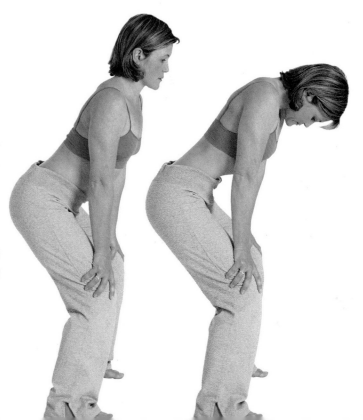

"Through the perfection of bandhas the yogi is able to lock himself into the 'eternal now,' devoid of the dualities of existence, motion, and change."
From *Moola Bandha, The Master Key* by Swami Buddhananada.

Jalandhara Bandha: throat lock

This seal slows down and acts as a channel for your breath, creating the soft, sibilant sound associated with *ujjayi* breathing (see page 9). It helps lower your heart rate, moderate your blood pressure, enhance your endocrine (hormonal) system, and calm your mind. The physical action also stretches your neck, stimulates the spinal cord, and removes tensions at the base of your skull.

Jalandhara practice

The Bridge pose (see below) is a good posture in which to practice *jalandhara bandha*. Lie on your back, bend your knees with your feet hip-width apart, press your palms into the floor, and lift your pelvis off the floor. Aim to create a diagonal line with your body from your shoulders through to your knees. To harness *jalandhara bandha*, contract your throat gently by swallowing to connect with the muscles at the back of your throat. Then continue to squeeze these muscles to narrow your air passage

and to create an internal echo on breathing. Pressing your chin against the notch at the top of your chest will help you do this. Take five deep *ujjayi* breaths. Then exhale, release the pose, and hug your thighs into your abdomen. Repeat this three times.

Mula Bandha: perinneal lock

This lower seal is the conscious muscular contraction of the perineum (cervix in women), which is situated between your anus and your genitals. The action of this lock balances both your hormonal system and your nervous system, due to nerve fibers that emerge from the pelvic area of the spinal cord.

Mula practice

It is essential to practice this *bandha* because differentiation between the three muscle groups in the pelvic floor is not easy at first. *Mula bandha* must be a lifting of the pelvis not of the anus or the

urogenital muscle. There are no specific yoga postures in which this can be practiced, so try each of the three contractions in turn to learn how each one feels. Contraction of the muscles in the urogenital area stops urination, contraction of the mucles in the anal area stops evacuation of the bowels, while *mula bandha* is a contraction of the area between the two.

INTEGRATING THE THREE LOCKS

Maha bandha is the contraction of all three locks together, which can be practiced in seated meditation at first. This is your ultimate aim: it will bring your yoga practice onto another level.

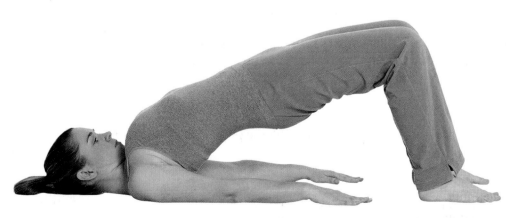

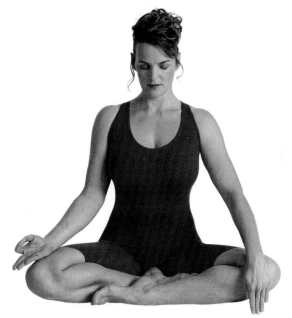

How to Practice

The full sequence of postures in this book takes approximately one and a half hours to complete, depending on your pace and energy level. However, it is not always possible to spend this long on your practice. It is more beneficial to do a short practice regularly than to do a huge session every now and then. A variety of shorter yoga programs based on the postures within this book are provided below.

HOW OFTEN?

Three times a week is a good initial goal for your yoga practice, but bear in mind that ideally you should practice daily in order to gain maximum benefit from the postures. As you progress, gradually increase the frequency and length of your sessions.

THE IMPORTANCE OF LOVING KINDNESS

It is crucial to monitor and adjust your practice according to your energy levels. Never strain yourself, and always pay great attention to what you are doing and how you feel each day, striving to free yourself of all harsh

expectations. This is an integral part of practicing what Buddhists call *metta*—loving kindness—toward yourself and others.

PACE YOURSELF

Five deep *ujjayi* breaths are advised in each posture but you may want to start with eight until you get used to the movements. If a posture becomes too challenging, don't be afraid to modify it according to the Confidence Builder provided on the top page. And if you feel tired at any point, adopt the rest

Be gentle and loving with your own mind and body just as you would be if adjusting someone else in a yoga posture.

WHAT YOU WILL NEED

All you need to practice *astanga vinyasa* yoga is yourself, a yoga mat, some energy and focus, and a peaceful place with enough space for you to stretch your body to its full height when standing and to its full length when lying down.

The area in which you choose to practice should be pleasantly warm, with good ventilation, and you should wear light or stretchy clothes so that your body feels unrestricted when moving. Please note that you should never perform yoga on a full stomach: it is advisable to leave at least two hours between eating and practice. The ideal time is first thing in the morning, before you have had your first food of the day.

posture shown on the relevant chapter opener. Hands-on adjustments shown on the top page of each exercise draw attention to areas of the body that may be hard to move into correct alignment or full position. Annotation is also provided to highlight additonal postural and alignment points. Strive to integrate these points into your practice, but do not let them override your sense of calm and focus throughout the postures.

Short Sequences

If the full one-and-a-half hour sequence in this book is too long, choose one of the shorter sequences below instead, according to your energy level and how busy you are at the time. When practicing Sun Salutation A, either after The Tree in the 20–25 minute practice or after Lord of the Dance in the 30–40 minute practice, link it smoothly to the next posture by jumping through from Downward Dog to Seated Staff at the end. If you choose the 30–40 minute practice, carry out a Half Vinyasa between each seated posture, starting after Seated Staff to Forward Bend and finishing after Seated Twist. Leave out the Half Vinyasa if you feel tired at any point.

5–10 MINUTE PRACTICE

Yogic Seal
    (pages 88–89)
Final Relaxation
    (pages 92–93)

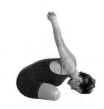

Yogic Seal

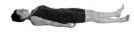

Savasana

20–25 MINUTE PRACTICE

Sun Salutation A: x 3
    (pages 16–21)
Sun Salutation B: x 1
    (pages 24–27)
Standing Forward Bends
    (pages 30–31)
Triangle
    (pages 32–33)
Wide-legged
    Forward Bends
    (pages 42–43)
The Tree
    (pages 52–53)
Sun Salutation A x 1
    (pages 16–21)
Shoulderstand
    (pages 80–81)
The Fish
    (pages 84–85)
Yogic Seal
    (pages 88–89)
Final Relaxation
    (pages 92–93)

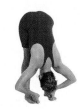

Standing Forward Bends

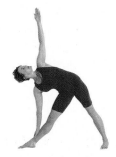

Triangle

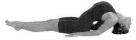

The Fish

30–40 MINUTE PRACTICE

Sun Salutation A: x 3
    (pages 16–21)
Sun Salutation B: x 2
    (pages 24–27)
Standing Forward Bends
    (pages 30–31)
Triangle
    (pages 32–33)
Side-angle posture
    (pages 36–37)
Twisting Side-angle
    posture
    (pages 38–39)
Wide-legged
    Forward Bends
    (pages 42–43)
Leg Raises
    (pages 48–49)
Lord of the Dance
    (pages 50–51)
Sun Salutation A x 1
    (pages 16–21)
Seated Staff to
    Forward Bend
    (pages 66–67)
Head to Knee posture
    (pages 68–69)
The Locust
    (pages 70–71)
Seated Twist
    (pages 74–75)
Shoulderstand
    (pages 80–81)
The Fish
    (pages 84–85)
Yogic Seal
    (pages 88–89)
Final Relaxation
    (pages 92–93)

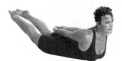

Twisting Side-angle posture

Seated Staff to Forward Bend

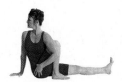

Head to Knee posture

The Locust

Seated Twist

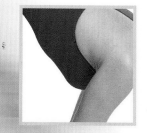
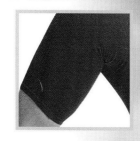
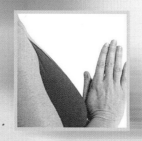
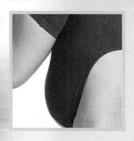
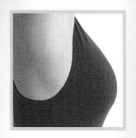
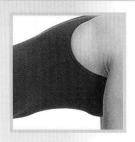

> *"If your mind is not clouded by unnecessary things, This is the best season of your life."*
>
> From the Mumonkan, an ancient Buddhist text

The Sun Salutation A sequence cultivates fitness, strength, alignment, and flexibility, and is traditionally practiced at dawn to welcome each rising sun. Carry out this flowing sequence at the beginning of your yoga session to warm up your body, engage your concentration, powerfully tone your muscles, and clear your mind for the practice to come.

The Mountain posture that starts and ends the Sun Salutation—*Tadasana*—forms the foundation for your practice. This pose is the first classical yoga posture cultivating alignment awareness, and giving you a sense of grounding through your feet, coupled with a sense of upward reach through your torso and head.

Start by practicing three sequences in a row, and build this up to five rounds as you progress. Remember to enter, inhabit, and exit all postures with seamless attention to your breath.

If the sequence becomes too challenging, rest momentarily by hanging in a loose forward bend pose: position your feet hip-width apart, slowly bend forward, place each hand on your opposite elbow to lightly fold your arms, and relax your arms, neck, and head until you feel restored and ready to continue.

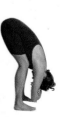

Sun Salutation A:Part 1

The starting pose for Sun Salutation A is Mountain (*Tadasana*), where you stand tall and steady as a mountain to cultivate a state of "attention without tension." This promotes good body awareness, correct alignment, and the focus of positive intention, in preparation for all the other postures. Once your feet and legs are firmly grounded in Mountain, you reach your torso and arms skyward into Raised Mountain (*Tadasana Urdhva Hastasana*), strengthening the joints and muscles in your legs, feet, arms, and hands. Next, you flow into a Forward Bend (*Uttanasana*), which brings oxygenated blood to your brain, massages your abdomen, further strengthens your legs, and stretches the whole back of your body. And the final step included on this page involves lifting your chest and looking up from the Forward Bend, in preparation to continue the sequence on page 19 by jumping back into Four-limbed Staff. It is important to be steady, yet internally vibrant, within every posture and to flow as smoothly as possible from each pose to the next.

A Steady Gaze

Shift your gaze smoothly between postures: from straight ahead in Mountain, to your fingertips in Raised Mountain, to your nose in Forward Bend, to just in front of your feet when you bend your knees to jump back.

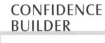

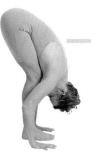

CONFIDENCE BUILDER

Bend your knees if necessary in the Forward Bend in order to rest your lower abdomen on your thighs, and to release your lower back.

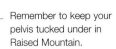

Remember to keep your pelvis tucked under in Raised Mountain.

Shift your biceps outward in Raised Mountain to help straighten your raised arms, and to drop your shoulders away from your ears.

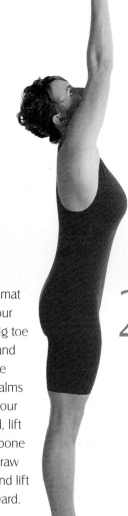

1 Stand at the front of your mat in Mountain by placing your feet together, with your big toe joints, inner ankle joints, and inner heels touching. Place your arms at your sides, palms facing your thighs. Press your feet firmly into the ground, lift your arches, tuck your tailbone under, open your chest, draw your lower belly inward, and lift the top of your head skyward.

2 *Inhale*, raise your arms above your head into Raised Mountain, keeping your arms as straight as possible. Press your palms together, look up without crooking your neck, and keep your tailbone tucked under.

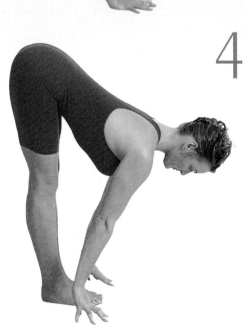

3 *Exhale*, hinge from the front of your hips into a deep Forward Bend, lowering your arms by drawing a wide circle with them, as if diving in slow motion. Place your hands on the floor beside your feet if possible. Drop your head and fully relax your neck.

4 *Inhale*, lift your chest and head, keeping your neck in line with your spine, straightening your arms and drawing in your abdomen, in preparation for jumping back to Four-limbed Staff.

Suryanamaskara

Sun Salutation A: Part 2

The energy-giving Sun Salutation is continued by jumping or lightly stepping back into the Four-limbed Staff (*Chaturanga Dandasana*). Here, you suspend the weight of your body on your palms and the base of your toes, developing strength in your upper body, abdomen, and legs. The flow into Upward Dog (*Urdhva Mukha Svanasana*) stretches your spine, cultivating strength and flexibility, and expands your chest, enhancing lung capacity. This pose tones your shoulders, hips, and the entire back of your body, and nourishes your heart and lungs with oxygenated blood, soothing your mind. It also cultivates a feeling of vitality and clarity of mind, as does the next key posture—Downward Dog (*Ardho Mukha Svanasana*).

The Power of Visualization

As you lower your body to the floor in Four-limbed Staff, imagine that you become as straight as a plank.

CONFIDENCE BUILDER

If jumping back to Four-limbed Staff is too difficult, simply step back one foot at a time, keeping your arms straight. Then bend your elbows into the sides of your rib cage and lie in a face-down position with just your knees, thighs, and abdomen lifted off the floor. Soon you will be able to lift your chest too.

Press your palms and feet firmly into the ground in Downward Dog, keeping your head down, and straightening your back as much as possible.

It is crucial in Downward Dog to draw in your abdomen and to lift up your sitting bones as high as possible.

FLOW IN

*From looking up in Forward Bend, **inhale**, press your hands firmly beside your feet, transfer your weight onto your hands, and lightly jump both feet back, raising your hips high as you do so.*

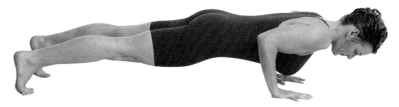

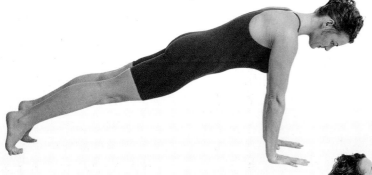

1 You should land at an angle to the floor in what is known as Diagonal Plank position, with your weight on your toes, your spine and arms straight, and your feet hip-width apart.

2 **Exhale**, bend your arms, and lower your body into Four-limbed Staff, hovering parallel above the floor on the palms of your hands and the balls of your feet. Your feet should be hip-width apart with your toes tucked under, and your palms pressed into the floor beside your rib cage, not your shoulders. Do not let your pelvis dip toward the floor or protrude upward. Keep your spine as straight as possible.

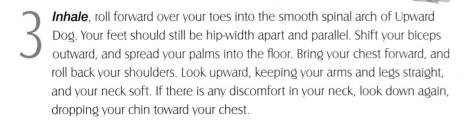

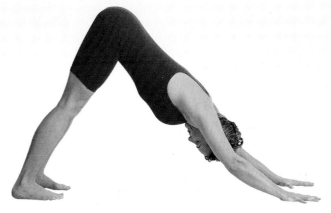

3 **Inhale**, roll forward over your toes into the smooth spinal arch of Upward Dog. Your feet should still be hip-width apart and parallel. Shift your biceps outward, and spread your palms into the floor. Bring your chest forward, and roll back your shoulders. Look upward, keeping your arms and legs straight, and your neck soft. If there is any discomfort in your neck, look down again, dropping your chin toward your chest.

4 **Exhale**, roll smoothly onto the balls of your feet, pushing your hips in the air to form an inverted "v-shape" with your body in Downward Dog. Your hands should remain shoulder-width apart, your feet hip-width apart, and your arms, legs, and spine as straight as possible. Point the middle finger of each of your hands forward, fully relax your neck, and press your hands and feet firmly into the mat.

• *Take 5 deep ujjayi breaths.*

Suryanamaskara

Sun Salutation A: Part 3

This final part of Sun Salutation A sequence brings you full circle, springing lightly through from Downward Dog to Forward Bend in order to return via Raised Mountain to where you first started—in Mountain. The *vinyasa* (breath-connected) jump through to Forward Bend is at the heart of this flowing sequence as it allows you to cultivate "energetic lightness," a quintessential component of enriching yoga practice. The Forward Bend brings oxygenated blood to your brain, and stretches the back of your body. Raised Mountain continues the dual sensations of grounding and transcendence that you experience in your jump-through. Mountain (*Tadasana*) returns you to the beginning, but this time with your hands in *namaste* position, the universal peace *mudra*— a calming gesture with which to complete your opening sequence.

Mindful Breathing

Direct your breath toward your heart as you end the sequence in Mountain with your palms pressing together. This creates a sense of peace and tranquility within you for the rest of your day.

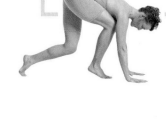

CONFIDENCE BUILDER

If springing through from Downward Dog to Forward Bend is too difficult at first, start by stepping your feet one at a time toward your hands.

Lift your hips as high as possible when jumping through from Downward Dog to Forward Bend, as if a harness attached around your pelvis is pulling them up. Also draw in your abdomen.

FLOW IN

From Downward Dog, **inhale**, *bend your knees, raise up onto tiptoe and look forward. Make sure to keep your hips high throughout.*

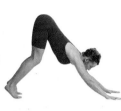

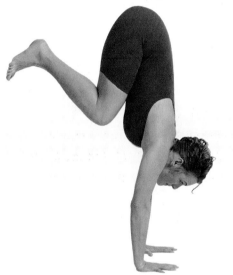

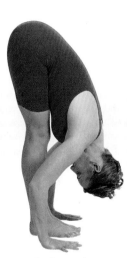

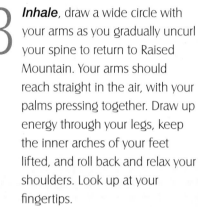

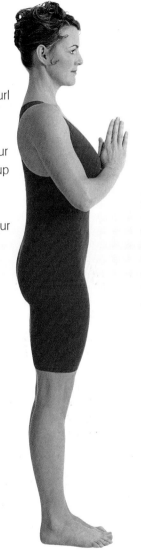

1 Briefly transfer all your weight onto your hands in order to spring both feet to the floor between your hands. As you jump, draw your hips above your shoulders before planting your feet together on the floor. This develops a slow, controlled lift, and a light jump performed with *uddiyana bandha* (see page 10).

2 On landing, **exhale**, and go into a deep Forward Bend, grounding your feet. Make sure that you release your neck and lengthen your spine as much as possible. Bend your knees to help you touch your abdomen to your thighs if you are experiencing any discomfort.

3 **Inhale**, draw a wide circle with your arms as you gradually uncurl your spine to return to Raised Mountain. Your arms should reach straight in the air, with your palms pressing together. Draw up energy through your legs, keep the inner arches of your feet lifted, and roll back and relax your shoulders. Look up at your fingertips.

4 **Exhale**, return to Mountain, bringing your arms to *namaste mudra*—prayer position (see page 7)—which helps you direct attention to your heart space, and in turn cultivate *bodhicitta* (positive emotional energy). Direct your gaze forward.

CHAPTER 2 SUN SALUTATION B

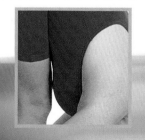 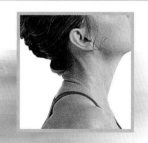 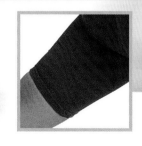 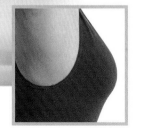 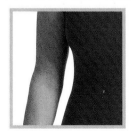 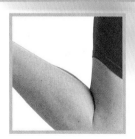

> # "To affect the quality of the day, That is the highest of Arts."
>
> By Henry Thoreau, a 19th-century writer

A development of the previous sequence, Sun Salutation B further cultivates your fitness, strength, alignment, and flexibility. Weaving two new poses—Fierce Pose and Warrior 1—into the sequence also helps you locate your center of gravity in the pelvis.

Fierce Pose stimulates your spine and opens your chest, while Warrior 1 opens and aligns your hips. The additional poses also draw attention to the symbolic union of opposites in yoga by deepening your sense of grounding from the waist down, while still encouraging you to reach toward the sky from the waist up.

Start by carrying out three sequences in a row and build up to five as you progress. It is important to learn the two new postures first, however, so practice moving between Mountain and Fierce Pose three times (see pages 24–25), and between Downward Dog and Warrior 1 three times (see pages 26–27), before integrating them into the full sequence.

If the sequence becomes too challenging, rest momentarily by hanging in a loose forward bend pose: position your feet hip-width apart, slowly bend forward, place each hand on your opposite elbow to lightly fold your arms, and relax your arms, neck, and head until you feel restored and ready to continue.

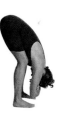

Sun Salutation B:Part 1

Suryanamaskara

This sequence interweaves two new postures into Sun Salutation A. The first of these postures, Fierce Pose (*Utkatasana*) replaces Raised Mountain from Sun Salutation A and is a powerful and challenging posture. The dynamic movement of opening your chest, reaching your arms skyward, and bending your knees as if sitting into an invisible chair strengthens your back, alleviates any stiffness in your shoulders, tones your internal organs, and strengthens your legs and ankles. It is a truly rejuvenating and empowering posture. Be sure to practice it several times on its own before weaving it into the Sun Salutation sequence. Raise your arms as straight as possible in the air without hunching your shoulders, and do not crook your neck.

The Power of Visualization

Imagine that you are moving through water to help you to gently synchronize the raising of your arms, the dropping of your hips, and the lifting of your gaze on the thread of your breath.

CONFIDENCE BUILDER

If the full Fierce Pose is too challenging at first, lock your chin onto your chest instead of looking up as you bend your knees, and clasp your hands behind you instead of stretching them in the air.

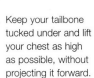

Keep your tailbone tucked under and lift your chest as high as possible, without projecting it forward.

Gently draw in your abdomen in Fierce Pose to create length between the pubic bone at the front of your pelvis and your sternum, so as to lift your rib cage and lengthen your spine.

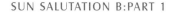

FLOW IN

Begin from Mountain with your hands by your sides (see Step 1 on pages 16–17).

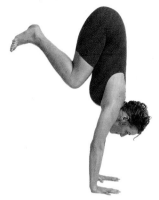

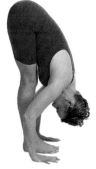

1 **Inhale**, bend your knees as if sitting into an invisible chair, and raise your arms straight above your head in Fierce Pose. Drop your hips, press your thighs together, tuck in your tailbone, and draw in your abdomen. This will maintain firm abdominal support to avoid over-arching your lower back. Press your palms together in the air, look up to your thumbs, and keep your shoulders relaxed.

2 **Exhale**, move smoothly into a Forward Bend, relaxing your head and neck, and bending your knees if necessary to let your abdomen touch your thighs.

3 **Inhale**, lift your chest and head from the deep Forward Bend, in preparation to jump back.

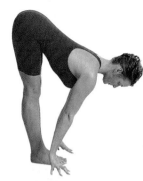

4 **Exhale**, transfer your weight to your hands and lightly spring or step back through Diagonal Plank to Four-limbed Staff (see page 19 for more detail).

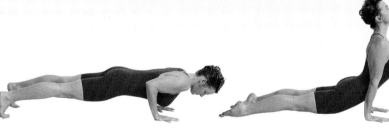

5 On landing in Four-limbed Staff, keep your feet hip-width apart, your elbows in tight beside your rib cage, and your body parallel to the floor. If this pose is too challenging, leave your upper body on the floor and only lift your kneecaps and thighs.

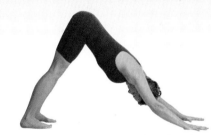

6 **Inhale**, move smoothly and gently through to Upward Dog, without over-arching your back or straining your neck.

7 **Exhale**, roll back onto the balls of your feet, and lift your hips skyward to flow into Downward Dog, pressing your heels into the floor if possible.

• *Take 5 deep ujjayi breaths.*

Sun Salutation B: Part 2

Warrior 1—or *Virabhadrasana* in Sanskrit—is the second new posture to be inserted smoothly into the Sun Salutation sequence. Named after the mythic Hindu warrior Virabhadra, this empowering posture strengthens your legs and spine, bringing flexibility to your knees, hips, and thighs. This pose also expands your chest and lungs, stretches your arms, relieves backache, and thoroughly cleanses your abdominal muscles and organs. This pose is a particularly effective one in which to cultivate concentration, poise, and steadiness. As with Fierce Pose, it is useful to practice Warrior 1 (Flow In and Step 1 below) as an individual pose before incorporating it into the whole sequence.

Mindful Breathing

Use deep, relaxed *ujjayi* breathing to help you find "effortless effort," and to appreciate the feeling of energy running through your limbs as you practice, like waves washing through you.

Concentrate on the alignment of your hips in Warrior 1, so that they both face the same direction as the foot of your bent leg.

CONFIDENCE BUILDER

If the full Warrior 1 pose is too difficult at first, practice it with your back foot pointing the same direction as your hips, and your back heel lifted off the ground to facilitate hip rotation. Then clasp your hands behind your back, and lock your chin onto your chest to release your shoulders and neck.

Keep your back leg as straight as you can, and firmly anchor your back foot to avoid tipping your weight forward.

FLOW IN

Inhale, *turn in the heel of your left foot by 15 degrees, bring your right foot between your hands, and bend your right knee to 90 degrees.* **Exhale**, *bring your torso upright, and place your hands on your hips.*

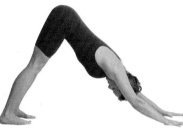

1 **Inhale**, raise your arms straight up above your head in Warrior 1, pressing your palms together in the air, keeping your spine straight, keeping your right knee bent at 90 degrees, and pressing your back foot firmly into the floor to keep equal weight through both feet. Direct your gaze to your thumbs.

2 **Exhale**, bend over and place your hands on either side of your right foot. **Inhale**, return your right foot in line with your left. **Exhale**, lower your body to hover in Four-limbed Staff, or lie face down if you need to.

3 **Inhale**, return to the smooth arch of Upward Dog, lifting your chest, rolling back your shoulders, and looking upward.

4 **Exhale**, return to Downward Dog, lifting your hips high and pressing your heels down. Then repeat Flow In to Step 4, bringing your left leg forward in Warrior 1 instead of your right (Flow In and Step 1).

5 **Inhale**, bend your knees, move up onto your toes, and look forward. **Exhale**, jump your feet between your hands, raising your hips as high as possible as you do so. See Confidence Builder on page 20 if this is too challenging at first.

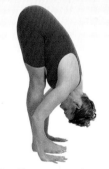

6 Flow into a deep Forward Bend on landing with your feet together from your jump-through. Fully relax your neck in this position.

7 **Inhale**, return to Fierce Pose, raising your arms straight in the air, bending your knees, and focusing your gaze beyond your hands.

FLOW OUT

Exhale, *return to Mountain with your hands in* namaste *(see page 7).*

CHAPTER 3 STANDING POSTURES

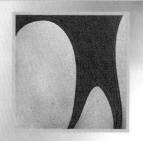 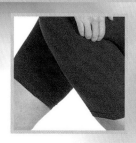 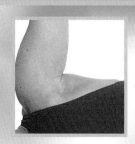 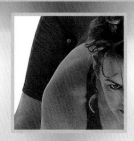 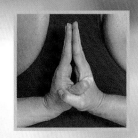 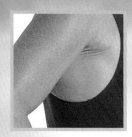

> *"Stand firm in that which you are. Do not run away."*
>
> By Kabir, a 15th-century mystic poet

Practice the standing postures in this chapter to deepen alignment awareness and develop and harmonize your qualities of strength, flexibility, and stamina. The range of stretches exercises your whole body by flexing, extending, laterally stretching, and twisting your spine. If you maintain full focus and awareness throughout the poses, they will bring power and good alignment to your legs, promote flexibility in your spine, and keep your joints fully mobile.

As in the Sun Salutation sequences, Mountain is the foundation posture so be sure to set it well (see page 7).

Traditionally, five breaths are taken in each full pose, as advised in this chapter. If this seems like too little at first, take eight breaths in each pose in order to inhabit each posture well, and avoid rushing your practice.

If the sequence becomes too challenging, rest momentarily by hanging in a loose forward bend pose: position your feet hip-width apart, slowly bend forward, place each hand on your opposite elbow to lightly fold your arms, and relax your arms, neck, and head until you feel restored and ready to continue.

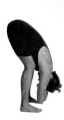

Padangusthasana—Padahastasana

Standing Forward Bends

The first of the standing postures, Forward Bends tone and stimulate your digestive system and liver. These poses also stretch the whole back of your body. They drain away any tension from your shoulders and upper back, provide your heart with an opportunity to rest, and feed your brain with fresh, oxygenated blood. The additional hand position in Step 4 deepens the practice. Relax your face entirely when in these postures, and allow your upper body to become soft like a rag doll.

The Power of Visualization

When bent over, imagine your spine is like a waterfall, with healthy energy pooling in the bowl of your skull.

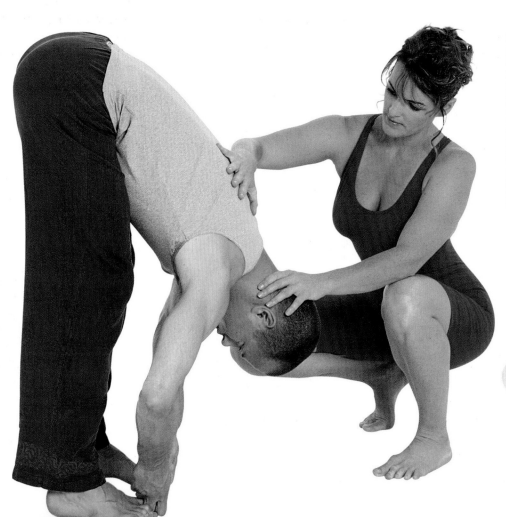

CONFIDENCE BUILDER

You can bend your knees if necessary in order to connect your abdomen to your thighs. Then hinge from the front of your pelvis.

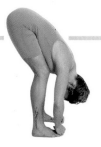

Don't hunch your shoulders or strain your back or neck when in the full pose. Relax your head and try to keep your neck in natural line with your spine.

FLOW IN

Inhale, position your feet to hip-width apart and parallel, place your hands on your hips, and then look up, opening your chest.

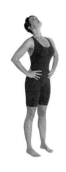

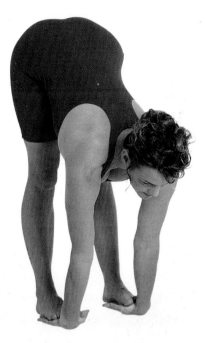

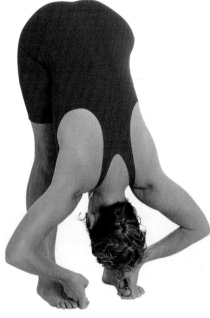

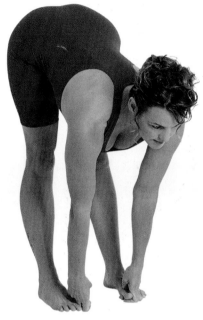

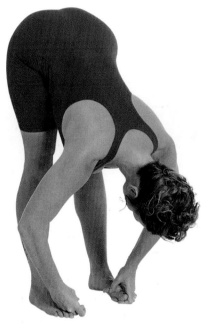

1 *Exhale*, hinge from the front of your hips into a fluid forward bend. Catch your big toes with the first two fingers of each hand.

2 *Inhale*, lift your chest and head to look forward. Lengthen the wall of your abdomen as much as possible—this prepares your spine to fold forward safely. Keep your palms facing each other.

3 *Exhale*, move your torso further over your thighs into a deeper forward bend, dropping and releasing your head.

•*Take 5 deep ujjayi breaths.*

4 *Inhale*, lift up your chest and head, draw in your abdomen, and look forward. Now place your hands beneath your feet so that the tips of your toes meet your inner wrists. *Exhale*, and repeat steps 1—3 with your hands in this new position. Then...

FLOW OUT

Inhale, lift your chest and look forward. *Exhale*, place your hands on your hips. *Inhale*, raise your torso up to standing and look forward.

Exhale, return to Mountain (see page 16–17).
Take one full breath.

Triangle

This classic standing posture aligns and energizes your spine from your tailbone through to the base of your skull. It exercises all joints, particularly within your spine, which is given a fantastic lateral stretch that alleviates backache. This posture strengthens your legs, hips, ankles, and feet, increases general flexibility, and cleanses and tones your abdominal and pelvic organs, relieving menstrual discomfort in women. Lift the inner arches of your feet when practicing this posture, pulling up through the inner seams of your legs to your groin.

The Power of Visualization

To open the front of your body, imagine a large inverted triangle with the top two points stretching from armpit to armpit and the bottom point touching just below your navel.

CONFIDENCE BUILDER

If the full posture is too difficult, try resting your hand on a yoga block, instead of on your leg, when bent over to the side. You also could leave the other arm on your side, so that you work the lower body only.

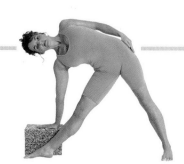

Fully open your upper body to expand your chest and abdomen. Pay particular attention to pulling back your top shoulder and hip.

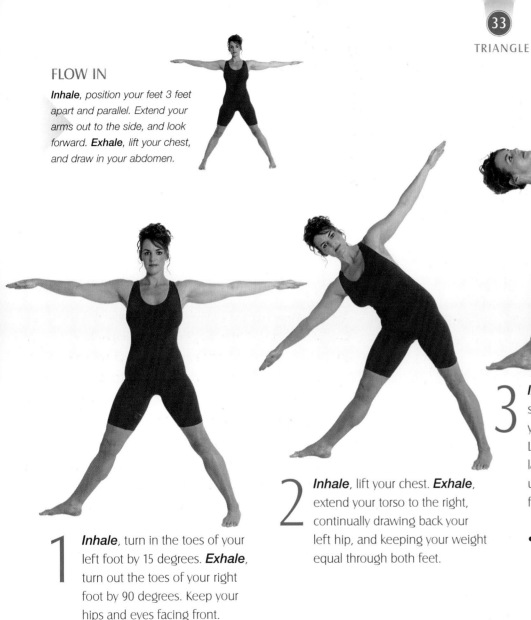

FLOW IN

Inhale, position your feet 3 feet apart and parallel. Extend your arms out to the side, and look forward. **Exhale**, lift your chest, and draw in your abdomen.

1 **Inhale**, turn in the toes of your left foot by 15 degrees. **Exhale**, turn out the toes of your right foot by 90 degrees. Keep your hips and eyes facing front.

2 **Inhale**, lift your chest. **Exhale**, extend your torso to the right, continually drawing back your left hip, and keeping your weight equal through both feet.

3 **Inhale**, open your chest. **Exhale**, stretch your left arm higher and reach your right hand toward your right ankle. Let your hand catch your leg wherever it lands on your leg, without letting your upper body close down or collapse forward. Look to your top hand.

•Take 5 deep ujjayi breaths.

4 **Inhale**, return to upright stance with legs apart and arms wide. **Exhale**, connect *uddiyana bandha* (see page 10). Next, reset your feet and hips— turn in your right foot by 15 degrees, turn out your left foot by 90 degrees, but keep your hips facing front—before repeating the posture (Steps 2 and 3) to the left side. Then...

FLOW OUT

*Inhale, return to standing upright, legs apart. Exhale, place your hands on your hips, ready for Twisting Triangle. **Take one full breath.***

Parivrtta Trikonasana

Twisting Triangle

Your body is now ready to progress to some deep-cleansing, twisting postures. The first of these—the Twisting Triangle—nourishes and strengthens your spine, tones and stimulates your internal organs, and massages your intestines. Twisting Triangle also strengthens your leg muscles, and thoroughly tones your hips. If you practice with abdominal awareness, it also helps to alleviate back pain. It is important to square both your hips to the side into which you are twisting.

The Power of Visualization

Pay particular attention to your neck as a continuing line of your spine, imagining it soft and long like a reed.

Keep your back foot firmly grounded in this posture.

CONFIDENCE BUILDER

Instead of the full posture, place your hand on your shin as you bend and twist, leaving your other arm on your lower back to create a deep rotation.

Try to get your spine parallel to the floor and to draw back your hip on the side into which you are twisting.

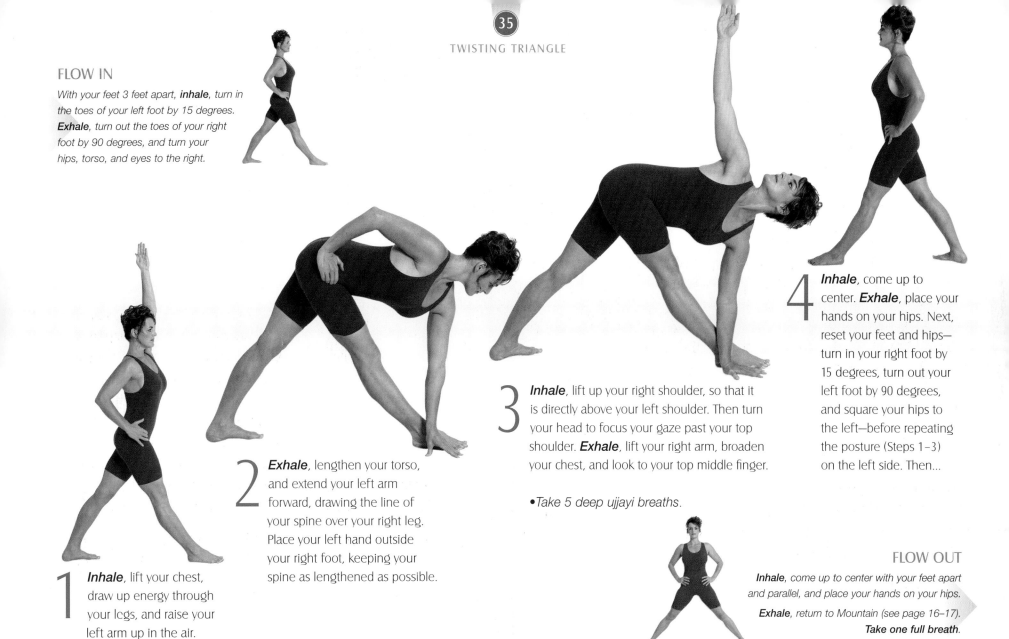

FLOW IN

With your feet 3 feet apart, **inhale**, turn in the toes of your left foot by 15 degrees. **Exhale**, turn out the toes of your right foot by 90 degrees, and turn your hips, torso, and eyes to the right.

1 **Inhale**, lift your chest, draw up energy through your legs, and raise your left arm up in the air.

2 **Exhale**, lengthen your torso, and extend your left arm forward, drawing the line of your spine over your right leg. Place your left hand outside your right foot, keeping your spine as lengthened as possible.

3 **Inhale**, lift up your right shoulder, so that it is directly above your left shoulder. Then turn your head to focus your gaze past your top shoulder. **Exhale**, lift your right arm, broaden your chest, and look to your top middle finger.

• Take 5 deep ujjayi breaths.

4 **Inhale**, come up to center. **Exhale**, place your hands on your hips. Next, reset your feet and hips—turn in your right foot by 15 degrees, turn out your left foot by 90 degrees, and square your hips to the left—before repeating the posture (Steps 1–3) on the left side. Then...

FLOW OUT

Inhale, come up to center with your feet apart and parallel, and place your hands on your hips.

Exhale, return to Mountain (see page 16–17). **Take one full breath**.

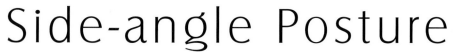

Side-angle Posture

This posture expands your chest, exercises your joints, and powerfully tones and strengthens your legs and the muscles in your back. The Side-angle posture also makes your hips and waist supple, and stimulates your abdomen, easing digestion through its vigorous internal massage. It also rejuvenates the abdominal organs, which is excellent for colonic health. It is important to keep your hips facing forward throughout.

A Steady Gaze

Focus your gaze on your top middle finger without crooking or tensing your neck, and keep every movement breath-synchronized.

Utthita Parsvakonasana

CONFIDENCE BUILDER

Instead of straining to get your hand on the floor, place your right forearm on your right thigh, bending your elbow. To open your chest deeply, wrap your left arm behind your back and catch your inner right thigh with your left hand.

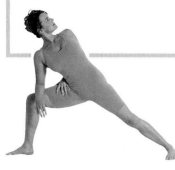

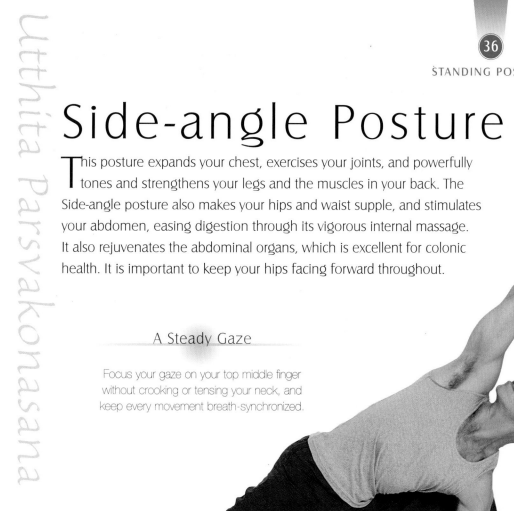

***Focus** on the diagonal stretch running through the whole top side of your body: lengthen from the waist down into the outside edge of your firmly-rooted foot, and from the waist up, through your top arm.*

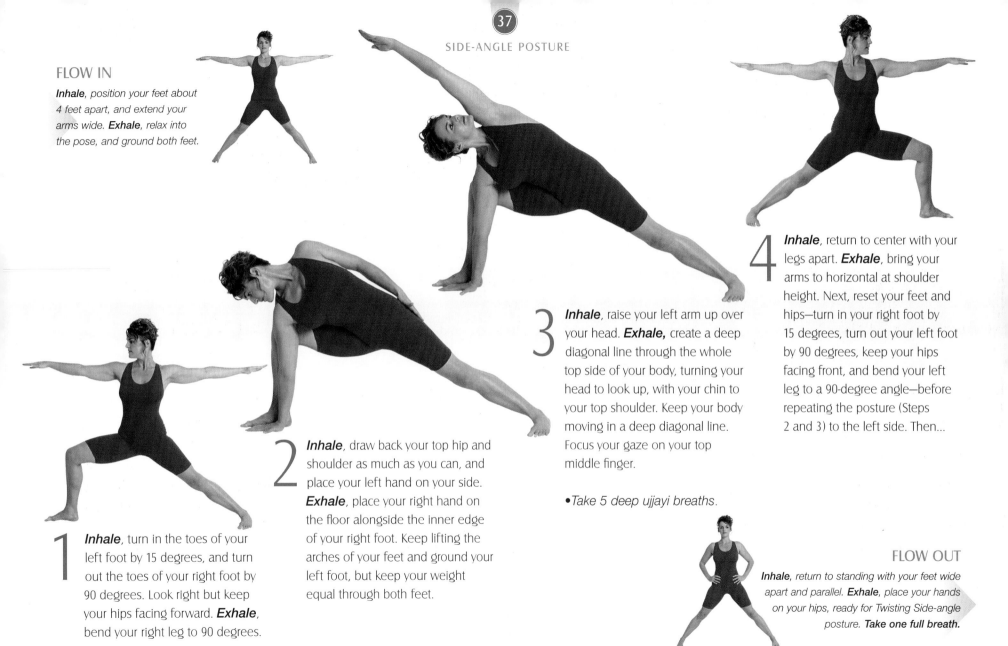

FLOW IN

Inhale, position your feet about 4 feet apart, and extend your arms wide. **Exhale**, relax into the pose, and ground both feet.

1 **Inhale**, turn in the toes of your left foot by 15 degrees, and turn out the toes of your right foot by 90 degrees. Look right but keep your hips facing forward. **Exhale**, bend your right leg to 90 degrees.

2 **Inhale**, draw back your top hip and shoulder as much as you can, and place your left hand on your side. **Exhale**, place your right hand on the floor alongside the inner edge of your right foot. Keep lifting the arches of your feet and ground your left foot, but keep your weight equal through both feet.

3 **Inhale**, raise your left arm up over your head. **Exhale,** create a deep diagonal line through the whole top side of your body, turning your head to look up, with your chin to your top shoulder. Keep your body moving in a deep diagonal line. Focus your gaze on your top middle finger.

•Take 5 deep ujjayi breaths.

4 **Inhale**, return to center with your legs apart. **Exhale**, bring your arms to horizontal at shoulder height. Next, reset your feet and hips—turn in your right foot by 15 degrees, turn out your left foot by 90 degrees, keep your hips facing front, and bend your left leg to a 90-degree angle—before repeating the posture (Steps 2 and 3) to the left side. Then...

FLOW OUT

Inhale, return to standing with your feet wide apart and parallel. **Exhale**, place your hands on your hips, ready for Twisting Side-angle posture. **Take one full breath.**

Parivrtta Parsvakonasana

Twisting Side-angle Posture

This posture is a more intense version of the Side-angle posture (see pages 36–37). It aligns and relieves any pain in your shoulders, back, and hips, and strengthens your legs and knees. This dynamic twist from the *astanga vinyasa* series tones the front of your body and massages and cleanses your inner organs.

Using *uddiyana bandha* (see page 10) will encourage deeper rotation and the literal feeling of "wringing out the spine." You can choose to practice the full pose with straight arms (see Step 3 below), or with your hands in *namaste mudra* (see right and page 7), which is a little less challenging.

Mindful Breathing

Meditate on the ebb and flow of your breath for a clear, unclouded mind.

CONFIDENCE BUILDER

If the full posture is a strain, turn your back toes to face your hips, raise your back heel, place your knee on the floor, and adjust your arms to namaste mudra.

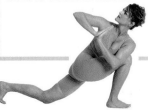

Whether practicing with straight arms or namaste mudra, aim to keep your chest lifted away from your pelvis. This creates space in your abdominal area to cleanse your internal organs.

You can either keep your back foot grounded at a 15-degree angle (see left), or turn it in by 90 degrees and lift your heel completely off the floor to help you square your hips (see Step 2 below).

FLOW IN

With your feet 4 feet apart, **inhale***,
turn in the toes of your left foot by
15 degrees.* **Exhale***, turn out the toes
of your right foot by 90 degrees, and
turn your hips and gaze to the right.*

1 **Inhale**, lift your chest, roll back
your shoulders, and harness
uddiyana bandha. **Exhale**, bend
your right leg to an angle of 90
degrees, drawing your right hip
back and your left hip forward.

3 **Inhale**, open your right shoulder, and reach
your right arm over your head. **Exhale**, create
a straight diagonal line with your right arm
along the right side of your body. Focus
your gaze on your top middle finger.

• *Take 5 deep ujjayi breaths.*

2 **Inhale**, lift your torso and twist to the right,
raising your back heel off the floor, and
easing the outside of your left arm
over your right thigh. **Exhale**,
straighten your left arm so
that your hand is on the
floor alongside the outer
edge of your right foot.

4 **Inhale**, straighten your right leg
and come up to center. **Exhale**,
place your hands on your hips.
Next, reset your feet and hips—turn
in your right foot by 15 degrees,
turn out your left foot by 90
degrees, and turn your hips to face
left—before repeating the posture
(Steps 1–3) to the left side. Then...

FLOW OUT

*Inhale, straighten your left leg, and come up
to standing, with your feet apart and parallel.*

Exhale*, return to Mountain (see page 16–17).*
Take one full breath.

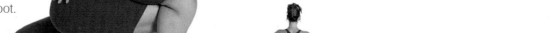
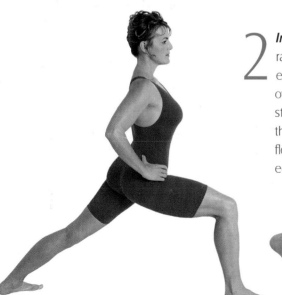

Ardha Chandrasana

Half-moon

The Sanskrit name of this graceful and stress-relieving pose—*Ardha Chandrasana*—reflects the body's resemblance to a crescent moon. The balance and coordination required make it an advanced pose, so practice it only if you are already confident in the Triangle pose. This pose stretches your spine and surrounding muscles intensively, helping to relieve any backache, while toning your stomach, massaging your internal organs, strengthening your knees, and improving general flexibility, circulation, alignment, balance, and concentration. You may need to rest your fingertips or hand on a yoga block for this posture so that your spine is parallel to the floor when in full position. Do not practice this pose if you have a severe headache, heart problems, or if you are tired.

CONFIDENCE BUILDER

If you feel that the full posture is too difficult, practice with your head facing forward, your standing leg slightly bent, and your upper arm resting along your upper thigh.

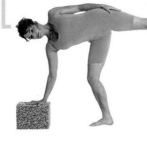

***Draw** back your top shoulder and top hip to keep your body as two-dimensional as you can and to expand the front side of your body.*

A Steady Gaze

Once you feel confident, look beyond your outstretched hand toward the sky.

FLOW IN

Inhale, position your feet 3 feet apart, and raise your arms to the sides. *Exhale*, turn in the toes of your left foot by 15 degrees, turn out the toes of your right foot by 90 degrees, keep your hips facing forward, and turn your head to the right.

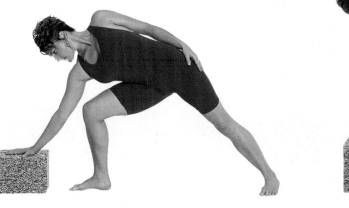

1 *Inhale*, draw up your torso. *Exhale*, bend your right knee, and place your right hand on the floor or on a yoga block in front of your right foot. Keep the left side of your body open.

2 *Inhale*, draw your body upward. *Exhale*, put your weight on your right foot and raise your left leg parallel to the floor below you. As you do so, straighten and stretch your right leg and arm as much as possible. Use your right hand for balance, and flex the foot of your raised leg.

3 *Inhale*, extend your left arm upward. *Exhale*, open your chest widely, and if you are comfortable, look up past your fingertips.

• Take 5 deep ujjayi breaths.

4 *Inhale*, bring your left arm down, and bend your right leg to plant your left foot on the floor. Stand with your feet 3 feet apart. *Exhale*, reset your feet—turn in your right foot by 15 degrees, turn out your left foot by 90 degrees, and keep your hips and gaze facing forward—before repeating the posture (Steps 1–3) to the left side. Then...

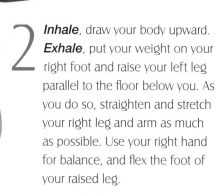

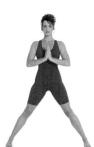

FLOW OUT

Inhale, bring your right arm down. *Exhale*, bend your left leg and come back up to standing center, with parallel feet and hands in namaste.

Exhale, return to Mountain (see page 16–17). **Take one full breath.**

Prasarita Padottanasana

Wide-legged Forward Bends

The literal translation from Sanskrit for this pose is "stretched out foot." These forward bends stretch your legs intensely, and rejuvenate your brain with fresh blood. Bends like these are also good recuperative poses to practice between dynamic standing poses, if needed. They align, rebalance, and soothe your mind and body by bringing positive calming energy to your heart and lungs, toning your internal organs, relieving any lower backache, exercising your hip and knee joints, and strengthening your legs. This pose can help to alleviate any tiredness or headaches you experience. If you have low blood pressure, make sure that you flow in and out of this pose very slowly.

CONFIDENCE BUILDER

If you experience any discomfort in your lower back when doing the full posture, bend your knees to make it more comfortable.

The Power of Visualization

Imagine colored petals are cascading down your spine, collecting in the bowl of your skull. Soften your neck and shoulders so that tension flows off you like water.

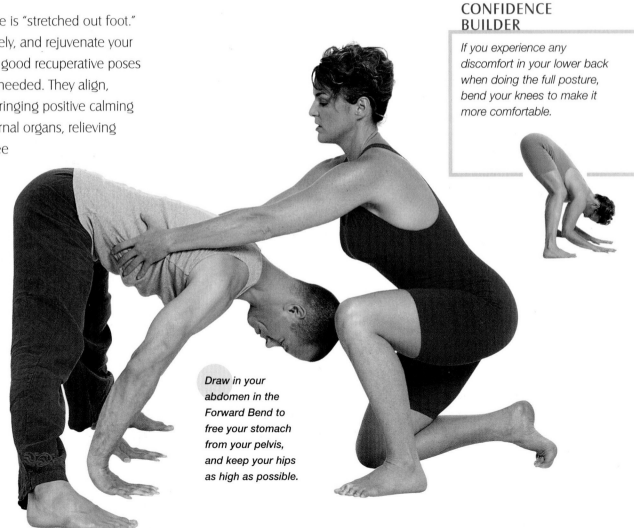

Draw in your abdomen in the Forward Bend to free your stomach from your pelvis, and keep your hips as high as possible.

FLOW IN

*Inhale, position your feet 3 feet apart, and extend your arms to the side. **Exhale**, pull in your lower abdomen to harness* uddiyana bandha.

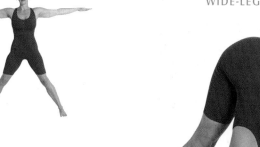

3 **Exhale**, move into a deeper forward bend, trying to place your head on the floor. Keep lifting your chest toward the floor to create space in your abdominal cavity. Relax and soften your shoulders and neck.

•*Take 5 deep ujjayi breaths.*

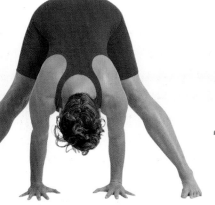

2 **Inhale**, look forward and draw in your abdomen. Lift your chest forward to keep the hollowing arch of *uddiyana bandha* (see page 10) in your abdomen.

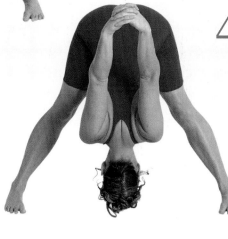

4 **Inhale**, lift your chest, look forward as in Step 2, and interlock your fingers behind your back. Next, **exhale**, look down, and move your head toward the floor again, extending your arms as far as possible toward the floor from behind your back.

•*Take 5 deep ujjayi breaths. Then…*

1 **Inhale**, lift your chest, and open your shoulders. **Exhale**, hinge from your hips into a forward bend. Place your palms on the floor between your feet, with your fingers pointing forward, and keeping your neck relaxed.

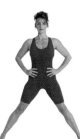

FLOW OUT

Inhale, slowly bring your torso to standing, lifting your chest, and placing your hands on your hips.

***Exhale**, return to Mountain (see page 16–17).*

Take one full breath.

Parsvottanasana

Intense Side Stretch

This movement opens up your chest and creates a sensation of deep expansion in your lungs, allowing you to feel strength and stability in your practice. Your lower body is rejuvenated, bringing flexibility to your legs, hips, and spine, the joints of your arms are toned, and your abdomen is massaged. *Parsvottanasana* also soothes your brain and can help ease pain in your neck, shoulders, elbows, and wrists. Keep rolling your shoulders away from your ears in this posture to enhance a feeling of openness in your chest and throat area. As always, lift the inner arches of your feet, broaden the balls of your feet, and spread your toes wide.

Mindful Breathing

Breathe deeply and freely, and concentrate on inhabiting the posture, sharing weight through both feet.

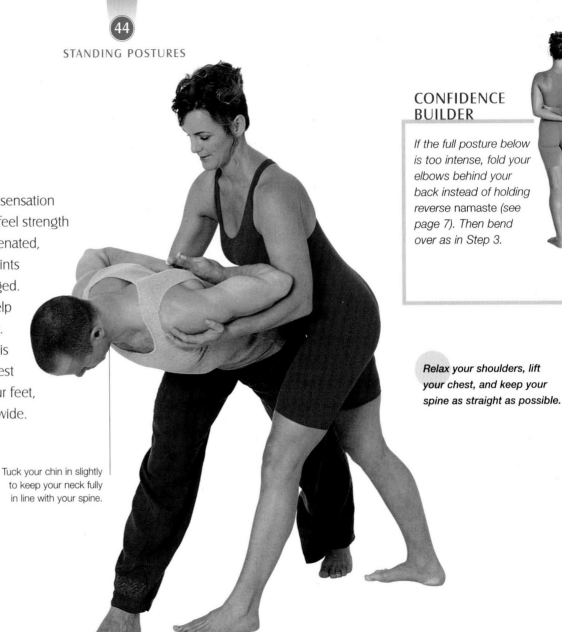

Tuck your chin in slightly to keep your neck fully in line with your spine.

CONFIDENCE BUILDER

If the full posture below is too intense, fold your elbows behind your back instead of holding reverse namaste (see page 7). Then bend over as in Step 3.

Relax your shoulders, lift your chest, and keep your spine as straight as possible.

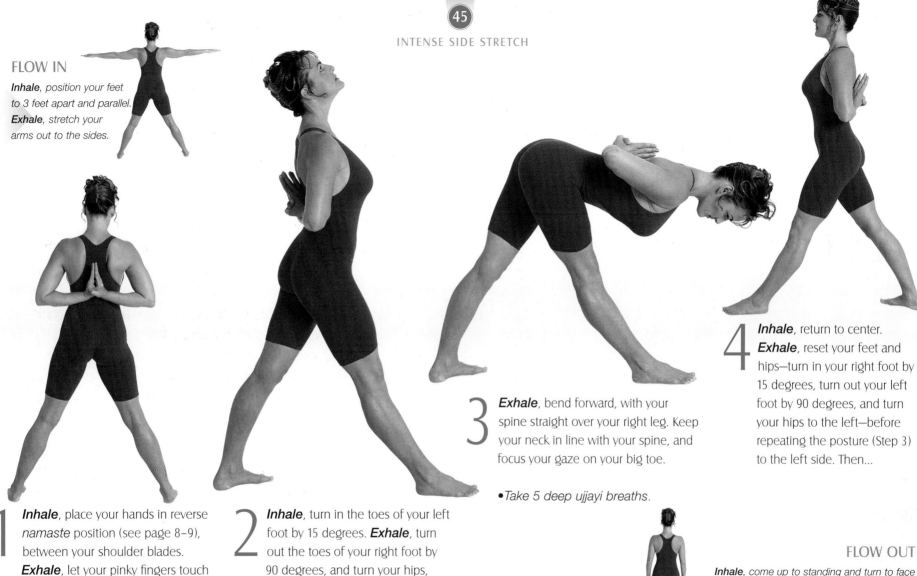

FLOW IN

Inhale, position your feet
to 3 feet apart and parallel.
Exhale, stretch your
arms out to the sides.

1 *Inhale*, place your hands in reverse
namaste position (see page 8–9),
between your shoulder blades.
Exhale, let your pinky fingers touch
your back, and keep your lower arms
horizontal. Don't hunch your shoulders.

2 *Inhale*, turn in the toes of your left
foot by 15 degrees. *Exhale*, turn
out the toes of your right foot by
90 degrees, and turn your hips,
torso, and gaze to the right, keeping
your hands in reverse *namaste*.
Inhale, lift your chest, and look up.

3 *Exhale*, bend forward, with your
spine straight over your right leg. Keep
your neck in line with your spine, and
focus your gaze on your big toe.

•*Take 5 deep ujjayi breaths.*

4 *Inhale*, return to center.
Exhale, reset your feet and
hips—turn in your right foot by
15 degrees, turn out your left
foot by 90 degrees, and turn
your hips to the left—before
repeating the posture (Step 3)
to the left side. Then...

FLOW OUT

Inhale, come up to standing and turn to face
forward, feet wide and parallel.

Exhale, return to Mountain (see page 16–17).
Take one full breath.

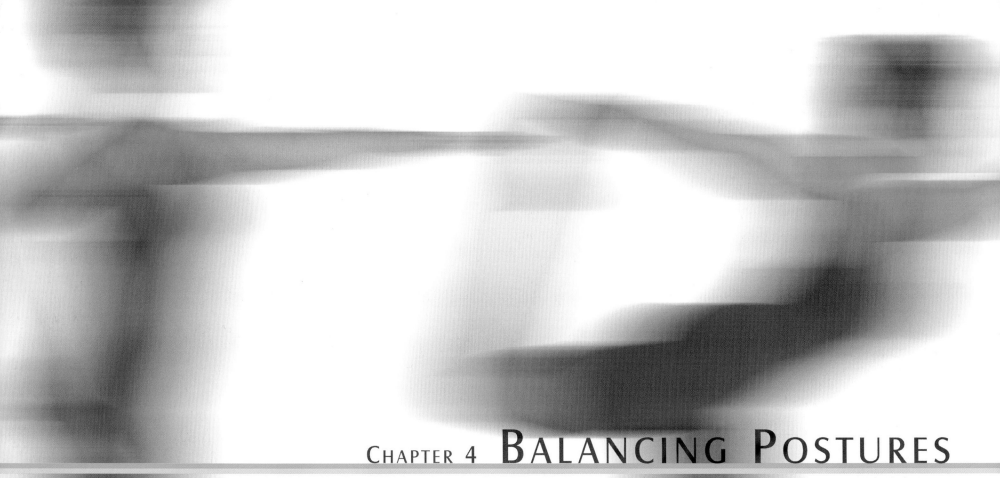

CHAPTER 4 BALANCING POSTURES

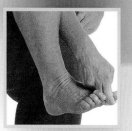 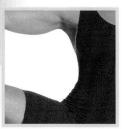 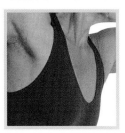 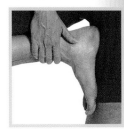 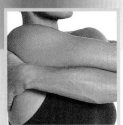 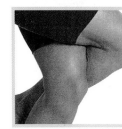

"*Act according to your true nature, in a balanced state…Being balanced, taking all things equally, this is yoga.*"

From Bhagavad Gita, core of the epic Hindu tale, The Mahabharata

Practice the balancing postures in this chapter to enhance the qualities of grounding, internal lightness, and grace within you. These poses explore the engaging tension between zeal and surrender, and between movement and resistance.

Striving to balance with "effortless effort" brings your attention to rest fully in the beauty and simplicity of the present moment, rather than projecting your thoughts into the future, or letting them fall back into the past.

Pay particular attention to maintaining a steady gaze when in the balancing *asanas*, looking toward an invisible horizon with a single focus.

If the sequence becomes too challenging, rest momentarily by hanging in a loose forward bend pose: position your feet hip-width apart, slowly bend forward, place each hand on your opposite elbow to lightly fold your arms, and relax your arms, neck, and head until you feel restored and ready to continue.

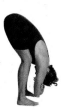

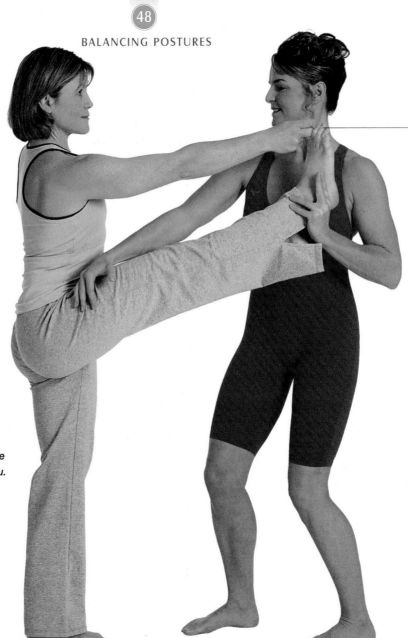

Utthita Hasta Padangusthasana

Leg Raises

This posture involves catching the big toe of your extended leg, in a challenging, focused balance. Your legs become strong and powerful, and, as with all balancing poses, your steadiness, grace, and poise are cultivated. Remember to maintain *uddiyana bandha* (see page 10) for firm abdominal support. This is essential in order to protect your lower back. It is also important to keep your standing foot well grounded—as if it has roots growing into the earth. To build alignment awareness in your hips, it is advisable to practice the Confidence Builder of this pose first (see right).

Try to keep your hips parallel when you raise your leg in front of you.

Mindful Breathing

Breathe deeply and freely to explore the quality of "attention without tension," as you balance on your standing leg.

Try to keep your leg as straight as possible, and spread the ball of your foot as much as you can.

CONFIDENCE BUILDER

This posture is very challenging, so if your lower back is under strain, or if the pose is too demanding, bend your lifting leg and clasp your knee or shin, firmly pressing your thigh to your lower abdomen.

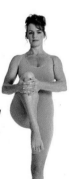

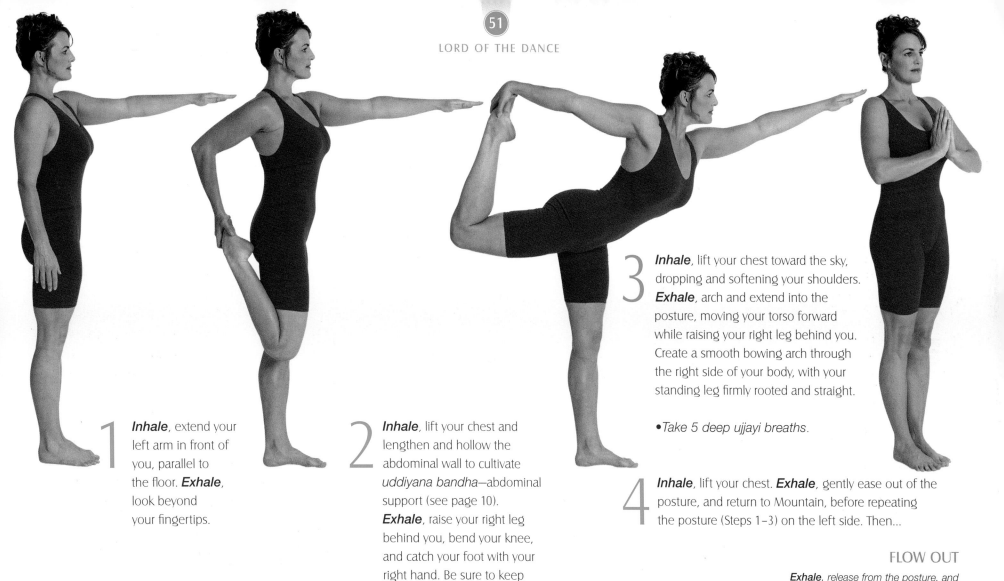

1 *Inhale*, extend your left arm in front of you, parallel to the floor. *Exhale*, look beyond your fingertips.

2 *Inhale*, lift your chest and lengthen and hollow the abdominal wall to cultivate *uddiyana bandha*—abdominal support (see page 10). *Exhale*, raise your right leg behind you, bend your knee, and catch your foot with your right hand. Be sure to keep your knees together.

3 *Inhale*, lift your chest toward the sky, dropping and softening your shoulders. *Exhale*, arch and extend into the posture, moving your torso forward while raising your right leg behind you. Create a smooth bowing arch through the right side of your body, with your standing leg firmly rooted and straight.

•*Take 5 deep ujjayi breaths*.

4 *Inhale*, lift your chest. *Exhale*, gently ease out of the posture, and return to Mountain, before repeating the posture (Steps 1–3) on the left side. Then...

FLOW OUT

Exhale, release from the posture, and return to Mountain (see pages 16–17). **Take one full breath.**

The Tree

You stand tall and firm in this posture, while balancing on one leg. The Tree increases lung capacity, and improves balance and steadiness, which brings increased awareness of good body alignment. This simple, calming pose also encourages you to appreciate the present moment and to become more at ease with everything around you, letting it flow on while you stand in stillness. Keep your tailbone slightly tucked under in this posture so that your torso sits well in your pelvic basin. Imagine that you are drawing up energy through your standing leg. It is also good practice to focus on the center of your brow during this pose, relating to the symbolic "third eye" of discernment, intuition, and perception. This leads to increased contemplation and stillness.

The Power of Visualization

Imagine that you are a plant reaching out of its flower bed, growing upward from your pelvis through your spine.

Keep your knee as wide as possible and your heel as high as you can on your inner thigh throughout this posture.

Relax your shoulders and lengthen the back of your neck, moving the crown of your head skyward.

CONFIDENCE BUILDER

If the full posture is too challenging at first, place your foot on the inside of your lower leg, rather than on your inner thigh. You can also choose to leave your hands on your hips at first.

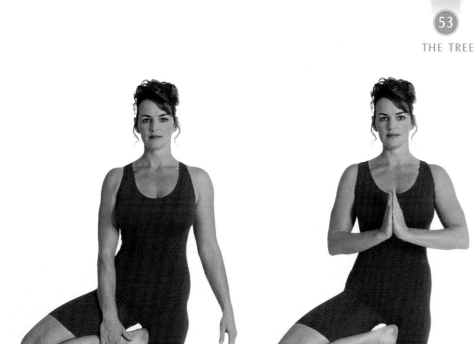

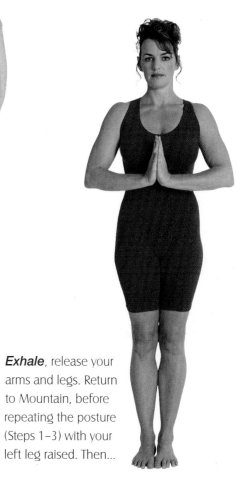

1 *Exhale*, root firmly into your left foot. *Inhale*, raise your right leg and plant your right foot as high as possible on your left inner thigh. *Exhale*, draw your right knee out to the right side, and keep your hips parallel.

2 *Inhale*, place your hands in *namaste* (see page 7), lifting your chest as you do so. *Exhale*, broaden your collarbones as you open from the center of your chest. Keep your tailbone tucked under.

•*Take 5 deep ujjayi breaths.*

3 *Inhale*, raise your arms straight up like an arrow, connecting your palms in the air, and drop your shoulders away from your ears.

•*Take 5 deep ujjayi breaths.*

4 *Exhale*, release your arms and legs. Return to Mountain, before repeating the posture (Steps 1–3) with your left leg raised. Then...

FLOW OUT

Exhale, release from the posture, and return to Mountain (see pages 16–17).
Take one full breath.

Garudasana

The Eagle

This calming posture is named after the king of birds because it requires the majestic strength and stature of an eagle. The Eagle pose involves intertwining your arms and legs in an intricate, one-legged balance, somewhat like a Celtic knot. This relieves tight shoulders, strengthens your ankles, and massages your legs. You require a steady focus and great determination to remain still in this posture with ease and lightness. Direct your breath into the back of your rib cage, and lift the base of your skull to lengthen the back of your neck. Tuck your tailbone under, relax your shoulders, keep your chin slightly tucked in, and maintain length in your abdomen, thus stretching your spine. Maintain a firm base for your standing leg by spreading your toes wide and broadening the ball of your foot, while continually lifting the inner arch of your foot.

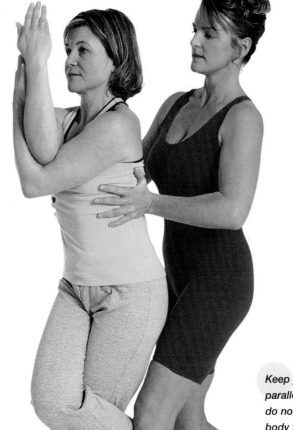

A Steady Gaze

As with all balancing postures, gaze with grace at one still point ahead in order to dwell in the present moment. This is known as *ekagra*.

Establish a very secure wrap with your legs—one foot hooked firmly behind your other calf—before introducing the arm wrap.

CONFIDENCE BUILDER

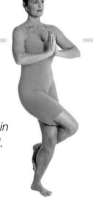

If the combination of arm and leg twists is too much for you at first, practice the leg-wrap with your hands in namaste at chest level.

Keep your hips parallel in this pose— do not allow your body to twist out of alignment.

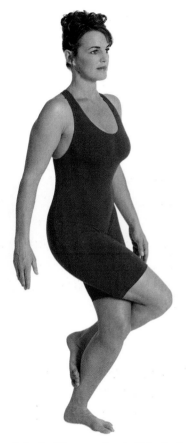

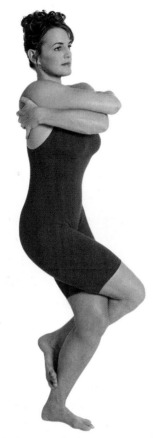

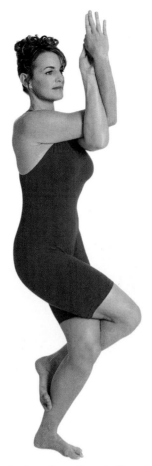

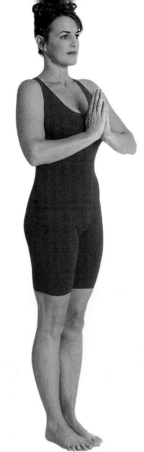

1 *Inhale*, lift your chest. ***Exhale***, bend both knees and wrap your right leg around your left leg, hooking the left calf muscle with your right foot.

2 ***Inhale***, wrap both arms around your shoulders—right arm over left arm— as if hugging yourself. ***Exhale***, aim for your hands to press on both shoulder blades, preparing your arms for the twist to come.

3 ***Inhale***, keep your legs in the same position, bring your forearms in front of you—your right elbow on top of your left, and wrap your arms around each other, aiming to join your hands in *namaste*.

•*Take 5 deep ujjayi breaths.*

4 ***Exhale***, release your arms and legs, and return to Mountain, before repeating the posture (Steps 1–3) on the left side. Then...

FLOW OUT

Exhale, *release from the posture, and return to Mountain (see pages 16–17).* **Take one full breath.**

CHAPTER 5 WARRIOR POSTURES

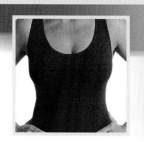
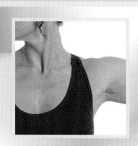
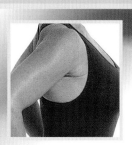
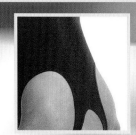
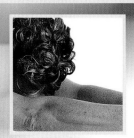
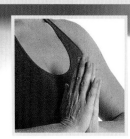

> " *Be one in self-harmony,
> in Yoga, and arise,
> great warrior, arise.* "

From Bhagavad Gita, core of the epic Hindu tale, The Mahabharata

Practice the three Warrior postures in this chapter to develop positive warrior qualities within you: focus, steadiness, and freedom from fear. These challenging postures also help you sit deeply in your pelvis, stretch freely up through your spine, and root deeply from your pelvis downward into your legs and feet.

Within this chapter, Warriors 1, 2, and 3 are taught as postures in their own right within a flowing sequence in order to help you practice them as correctly and as deeply as possible.

Warrior 3 explores the liberating feeling of an extended balance, cultivating a sense of grace and poise within you. But only practice this pose once you are very confident in Warriors 1 and 2, for it is taught in the advanced series in traditional *astanga vinyasa* yoga.

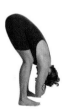

If the sequence becomes too challenging, rest momentarily by hanging in a loose forward bend pose: position your feet wide apart, slowly bend forward, place each hand on your opposite elbow to lightly fold your arms, and relax your arms, neck, and head until you feel restored and ready to continue.

Virabhadrasana

Warrior 1 to 2

It is said that to truly inhabit the Warrior postures is to exist purely in the present moment. Each pose increases knee and thigh flexibility, strengthens your spine, stretches your arms, and exercises your shoulder joints.

Each pose also opens your chest, increases lung capacity, and replaces tension around the heart with focused energy. You should not practice the Warrior postures if you have heart problems.

In the traditional *astanga vinyasa* sequence, Warrior 1 with your arms extended upward (see Step 2 below), is practiced with the right leg bent first and then the left, before progressing to Warrior 2 (see Step 3 below) first to the left and then to the right. However, the sequence is modified below for learning purposes.

The Power of Visualization

Imagine that you are sitting in a saddle. Also harness *uddiyana bandha* as if it is an invisible belt around your lower abdomen.

In Warrior 2 position (see left), stand as if the back of your body is touching a wall behind you. Keep drawing back the hip and shoulder on the side of your straight leg, aiming to keep weight equal through both feet.

CONFIDENCE BUILDER

If you experience any difficulty during Warrior 1, clasp your hands behind you and lock your chin onto your chest (see Confidence Builder on page 26) until you are ready to attempt the full posture with your gaze up. In Warrior 2, place your hands on your hips, instead of out to the side (see below).

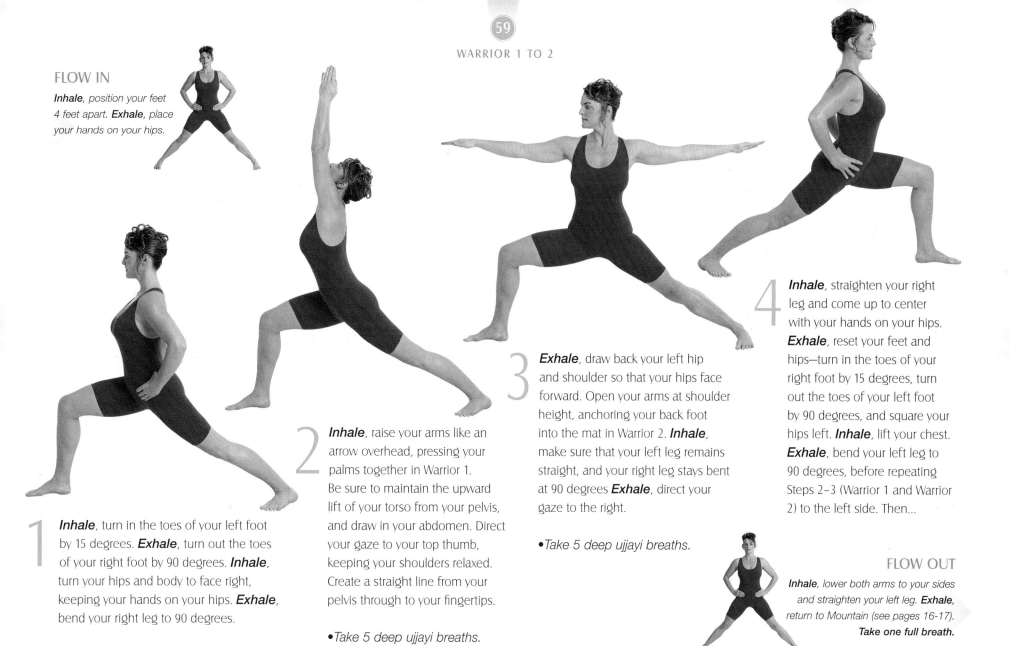

FLOW IN

Inhale, position your feet 4 feet apart. **Exhale**, place your hands on your hips.

1 **Inhale**, turn in the toes of your left foot by 15 degrees. **Exhale**, turn out the toes of your right foot by 90 degrees. **Inhale**, turn your hips and body to face right, keeping your hands on your hips. **Exhale**, bend your right leg to 90 degrees.

2 **Inhale**, raise your arms like an arrow overhead, pressing your palms together in Warrior 1. Be sure to maintain the upward lift of your torso from your pelvis, and draw in your abdomen. Direct your gaze to your top thumb, keeping your shoulders relaxed. Create a straight line from your pelvis through to your fingertips.

•Take 5 deep ujjayi breaths.

3 **Exhale**, draw back your left hip and shoulder so that your hips face forward. Open your arms at shoulder height, anchoring your back foot into the mat in Warrior 2. **Inhale**, make sure that your left leg remains straight, and your right leg stays bent at 90 degrees **Exhale**, direct your gaze to the right.

•Take 5 deep ujjayi breaths.

4 **Inhale**, straighten your right leg and come up to center with your hands on your hips. **Exhale**, reset your feet and hips—turn in the toes of your right foot by 15 degrees, turn out the toes of your left foot by 90 degrees, and square your hips left. **Inhale**, lift your chest. **Exhale**, bend your left leg to 90 degrees, before repeating Steps 2–3 (Warrior 1 and Warrior 2) to the left side. Then...

FLOW OUT

Inhale, lower both arms to your sides and straighten your left leg. **Exhale**, return to Mountain (see pages 16-17). **Take one full breath.**

Virabhadrasana

Warrior 3

An extension of the first two Warrior postures, Warrior 3 brings further strength to your legs, tones your abdomen, and cultivates balance, grace, and focus in your mind and body. This beautiful posture is an advanced and challenging one, so it should only be attempted once you are comfortable and confident in Warrior 1 and Warrior 2. Ultimately, you are aiming to put your spine and extended leg in a straight line, parallel to the floor. You may need stacked yoga blocks under your hands to help you achieve this. Omit Step 4 at first, leaving your hands on the floor for extra support.

The Power of Visualization

Once established in the pose, imagine that you are flying, with your arms extending forward and your raised leg extending away from you. Picture yourself being pulled in two directions: beyond your fingertips and beyond your toes.

It is important to keep your neck in a continuous line with your spine, so tuck your chin slightly toward your chest.

CONFIDENCE BUILDER

If the posture feels too challenging at first, place your hands on stacked books or yoga blocks to learn to balance with support. Do not attempt to lift your arms up until you are confident in this foundation.

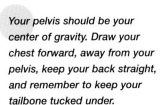

Your pelvis should be your center of gravity. Draw your chest forward, away from your pelvis, keep your back straight, and remember to keep your tailbone tucked under.

FLOW IN

Begin from Mountain (see pages 16-17).

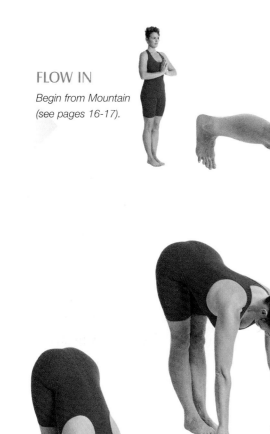

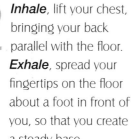

1 **Exhale**, move gently into a Forward Bend (see pages 30–31), relaxing your neck.

2 **Inhale**, lift your chest, bringing your back parallel with the floor. **Exhale**, spread your fingertips on the floor about a foot in front of you, so that you create a steady base.

3 **Inhale**, bend your left leg, and raise your right leg straight out behind you, parallel with the floor. **Exhale**, straighten your left leg to take the weight of your body. Be careful not to lock the knee of your standing leg.

• *Take 5 deep ujjayi breaths*.

4 Then, only if you are comfortable, **inhale**, lift your torso, and raise your arms forward in line with your whole body. **Exhale**, place your palms together, and be sure to harness *uddiyana bandha* (see page 10). If you are confident in this pose, direct your gaze forward past your fingertips. Make sure that you flex, rather than point, your raised foot.

• *Take 5 deep ujjayi breaths*.

5 **Inhale**, deepen the stretch. **Exhale**, slowly bring your arms and leg back to the floor. **Inhale**, gently come up to Mountain, before repeating the posture (Steps 1–4), this time raising your left leg behind you. Then...

FLOW OUT

Exhale, fold into a Forward Bend. *Inhale*, return to Mountain. **Take one full breath.**

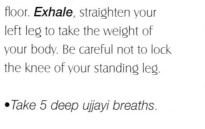

CHAPTER 6 SEATED POSTURES

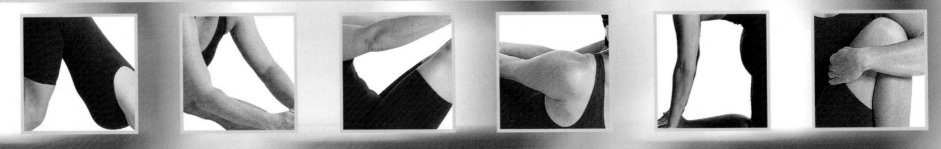

> " *Don't go outside to see the flowers my friend... Inside your body there are flowers... That will do for a place to sit.* "
>
> By Kabir, a 15th-century mystic poet

Practice the seated postures after the standing and balancing ones to stretch out your spine and exercise the joints in your legs through a combination of back-bending, forward-bending, and twisting. These poses free your hips, groin, and lower back, and connect you more firmly to the ground through your sitting bones.

The backbends (see pages 70–73) energize your body and remove any negativity. This can lead to unforeseen emotional releases, so practice these poses, in particular, with the Buddhist concepts of loving kindness (*metta*) and non-violence (*ahimsa*).

The linking sequence for the seated postures is the Half Vinyasa, which is shown in full on pages 64–65. Practice this sequence smoothly between each seated posture, as shown in the Flow Out. This encourages continuous movement with the breath, as well as the realignment of your spine, and the generation of a cleansing heat (*tapas*) within you.

If the sequence becomes too challenging, rest momentarily by lying on your back, and hugging your knees toward your chest. You can rock gently from side to side if you wish until you feel restored and ready to continue.

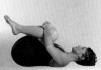

HALF VINYASA

This sequence contains many poses that will be familar to you from Sun Salutation A (pages 14–21), but they now begin and end in a seated position, providing a smooth, vital link between all the seated postures in this chapter. The Half Vinyasa sequence is at the heart of *astanga vinyasa* yoga, weaving your practice together into an unbroken flow of breath-connected movement, described by Guruji Sri K. Pattabhi Jois, a living master and teacher of *astanga vinyasa* yoga, as a "garland of postures." The light spring-throughs from Cross-legged position back to Four-limbed Staff (Steps 2–3, below) and then from Downward Dog into Seated Staff (Step 8, below) are challenging but worthwhile. Step through from one pose to the next until you build up the power and stamina over time to jump through. Move as smoothly as possible to flow every posture into the next.

CONFIDENCE BUILDER

Do not be disheartened if you cannot manage the full jumps at first, whether backward or forward. Press your hands into the floor, raise your hips as high as possible with your feet still on the floor, and step through one foot at a time.

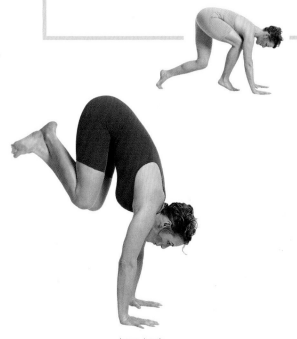

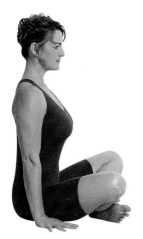

Cross-legged

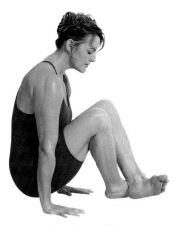

Cross-legged lift

Jump-back

1 **Exhale**, sit cross-legged, and place your hands firmly beside your hips.

2 **Inhale**, keep your knees high, and lift your legs into *Uth Pluthi* so that all your weight is on your straight arms.

3 Then harness *uddiyana* and *jalandhara bandha* to help you swing back from *Uth Pluthi*, raising your hips high and directing your feet behind you.

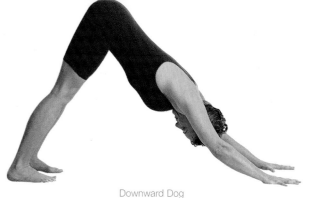

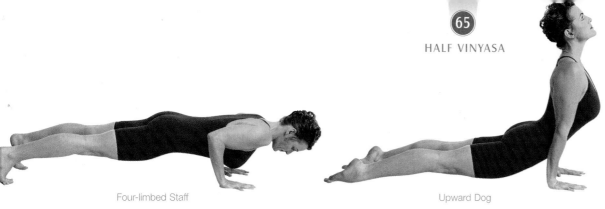

Four-limbed Staff

Upward Dog

Downward Dog

4 *Exhale*, land gently in Four-limbed Staff with your body parallel to the floor. Your legs should be straight, your feet hip-width apart, your toes tucked under, your arms bent at a 90-degree angle, and your palms pressed into the floor beside your rib cage.

5 *Inhale*, gently roll forward over your toes into Upward Dog, bringing the tops of your feet onto the floor and raising your upper body into a smooth spinal arch. Keep your arms and legs straight, open your chest, relax your shoulders, and look upward.

6 *Exhale*, roll back onto the balls of your feet, lift your sitting bones in the air, keep your arms and legs straight, and your palms pressed into the ground, and push your heels down into the ground to form Downward Dog. Keep your hands shoulder-width apart and your feet hip-width apart.

•*Take one deep ujjayi breath.*

Prepare to jump

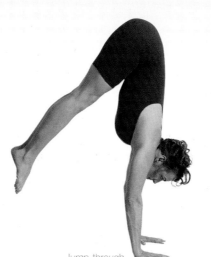

Jump-through

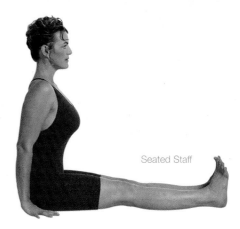

Seated Staff

7 *Inhale*, bend your knees, move up onto your toes, and look forward from Downward Dog.

8 *Exhale*, jump through to a seated position by lifting your feet behind you, raising your hips as high as you can and transferring all your weight onto your hands.

9 Slowly swing your legs through between your hands, and land in Seated Staff (see pages 66-67) as smoothly as you can.

Dandasana—Paschimottanasana

Seated Staff to Forward Bend

The Seated Staff—*Dandasana*—is the foundation posture for all the seated poses, just as Mountain is for the standing, balancing, and warrior poses. It is essential to do it properly by positioning equal weight through both buttocks, keeping your spine straight, your abdomen lengthened, and your chest lifted. *Dandasana* encourages good breathing and tones muscles in your chest, back, abdomen, and legs. This fine-tuning of your body is continued in the Forward Bend, which rests your heart and brain, and soothes your adrenal glands. This calming pose also has a massaging effect, which helps your digestion, and replenishes your bladder and reproductive organs.

Mindful Breathing

Expand your breath into the sides of your rib cage, contemplating its soothing, meditative sound—the pulse of your practice.

As always, it is important to lift your chest and draw in your abdomen, harnessing *uddiyana bandha*.

CONFIDENCE BUILDER

If the full Forward Bend is too intense at first, avoid straining your back by bending your knees slightly, and placing your hands on your shins instead of on your feet. This will help you press your lower belly toward your thighs.

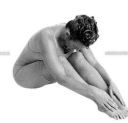

Be sure to relax your shoulders when in Seated Staff. Also lengthen the back of your neck by tucking your chin in slightly so that your spine is in natural alignment.

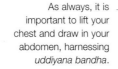

FLOW IN

Practice one Sun Salutation A sequence from Mountain through to Downward Dog (see pages 17–19). Then bend your knees and step or spring through into a seated position (see below).

1 Sit up tall with your legs stretched out in front of you and equal weight through both buttocks. Press the backs of your knees toward the floor, and flex your feet in this Seated Staff position.

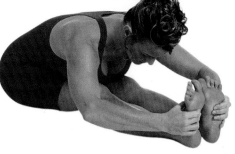

2 *Inhale*, lift your chest, and raise your arms above your head. *Exhale*, start to fold forward from the front of your hips, and catch your big toes with the first two fingers of each hand, keeping your neck in line with your spine. *Inhale*, lift your chest, and draw in your lower belly.

3 *Exhale*, lower yourself deeper into the pose, and direct your gaze toward your toes. Be sure to stretch from the base of your spine, and keep lifting your chest to massage your abdomen.

•*Take 5 deep ujjayi breaths*.

4 *Inhale*, look up, lift your chest, and hollow your lower belly, still with your fingers hooked around your big toes. *Exhale*, change the position of your hands by wrapping them around the outside edges of your feet. Then, lower yourself again into a deep but gentle Forward Bend.

•*Take 5 deep ujjayi breaths*.

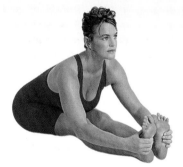

5 *Inhale*, look up from this position, lifting your chest. Then...

FLOW OUT

Return to Seated Staff. Then cross your legs to flow into the Half Vinyasa sequence (see left and pages 64–65). End by springing or stepping through from Downward Dog to Seated Staff.

Janu Sirsasana

Head to Knee Posture

This hip-opening posture soothes your brain and heart, tones your abdominal organs, and stimulates your digestive system. The Head to Knee posture also stretches and rejuvenates your spine, strengthens your legs and hips, and frees your lower back. With regular practice, your spine, shoulders, and hips re-align and become more flexible. This pose also tones your abdomen and exercises all your joints. Be careful doing this posture if you have any problems with your knees: do not continue if you experience any discomfort. To warm-up for this posture, cradle your leg in your arms and rock it gently from side to side to open the hip you are about to stretch.

The Power of Visualization

When extending forward, imagine water is falling onto and rolling off your upper back. This will allow your shoulders to soften and release.

Draw open your knee as wide as possible to unlock your hip joint. Then be sure to face your chest directly over your straight leg before gently bending forward into the pose.

CONFIDENCE BUILDER

If your knees feel at all vulnerable, place a tightly rolled towel in the hinge of your bent knee to take away some pressure. Then reach down for your lower leg instead of your foot.

It is important to flex the foot of your extended leg and to press the back of your knee into the ground.

FLOW IN

*Begin from Seated Staff
(see pages 66–67).*

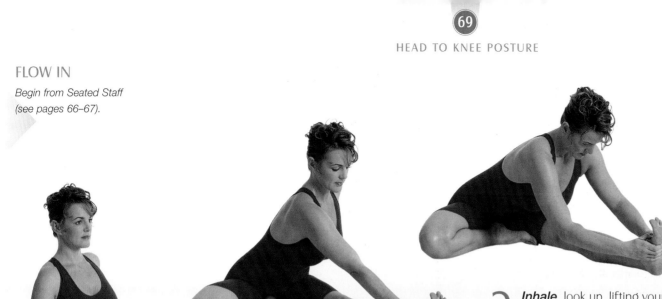

1 **Inhale**, bend your right knee and place it
out to the side, with your right foot touching
your left inner thigh. **Exhale**, position your
lifted chest in line with your left leg, leaving
your left hand on the floor behind you.

2 **Inhale**, raise your right arm overhead.
Then **exhale**, bend from the front of
your hips, extending your torso over
your straight left leg. Catch your left
foot with your right hand, leaving
your left hand on the floor.

•*Take 5 deep ujjayi breaths.*

3 **Inhale**, look up, lifting your chest, and
keeping your lower abdomen drawn in.
Exhale, fold deeper into the bend,
bringing your left hand to catch your left
foot, too. Press the back of your left knee
into the floor, stretch out the toes of your
left foot, and make sure you do not
round your back to achieve the bend.

•*Take 5 deep ujjayi breaths.*

4 **Inhale**, look up. **Exhale**,
come up from the forward
bend and straighten your
right leg to return to Seated
Staff. Next, repeat the
posture (Steps 1–3) on the
other side, starting from
the position above by
drawing back your left
knee. Then...

FLOW OUT

*Return to Seated Staff. Then cross your legs to
flow into the Half Vinyasa sequence (see left and
pages 64–65). End by lowering yourself from
Downward Dog to lie face-down on the floor.*

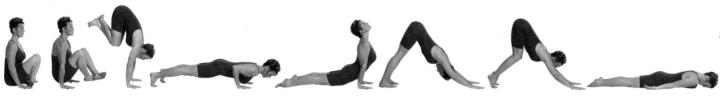

Salabhasana

The Locust

The Sanskrit word for locust—*Salabhasana*—is very fitting for this pose because the body takes on the form of a resting locust when in the full posture. Taken from the second series in the traditional *astanga vinyasa* yoga practice (see page 6), this elegant pose stretches and strengthens your lower back beautifully and safely, relieving lower back pain. It is wonderful preparation for deeper back bends, such as the Camel posture (see pages 72–73). The smooth arch of the posture not only tones the back of your body, but also exercises the front—massaging your stomach, stimulating digestion, and opening your chest to increase space around your heart and lungs. Take care not to strain your neck when practicing this pose.

The Power of Visualization

Imagine your spine arching smoothly through your body like the sweeping stem of a leaf after rain. Balance delicately on your navel.

Focus on lifting your chest forward and rolling back your shoulders. At the same time, stretch your legs straight back, making sure that you keep them firmly pressed together and point your toes.

CONFIDENCE BUILDER

If your neck feels in any way strained, look down instead of forward. And if you suffer from any back pain, practice with your thighs slightly apart and your legs bent at the knees, with your lower legs pointing upward.

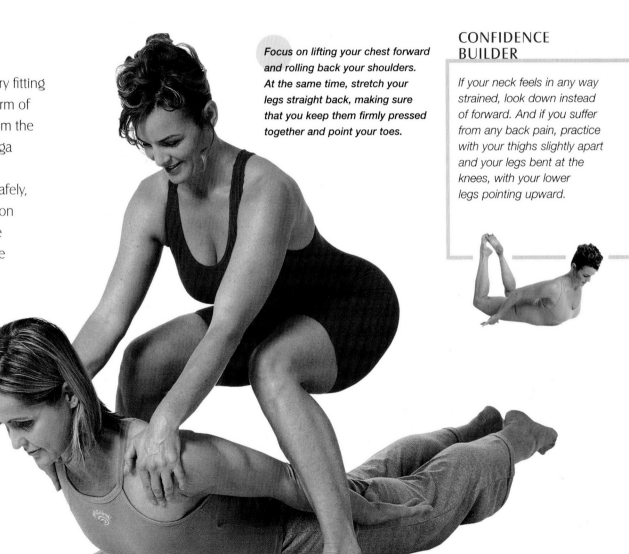

FLOW IN

Begin lying face-down, with your forehead touching your mat. Press your legs together, point your toes, and place your arms, palms-up, by your sides.

1 **Inhale**, raise your upper body into a deep, smooth arch, keeping your legs straight and pressed together on the floor. **Exhale**, gaze forward, lifting and broadening across your chest and collarbones, and rolling back your shoulders, Make sure that you keep your neck in line with your spine, and your hands, palms-up, on the floor.

2 **Inhale**, lift your legs off the floor behind you, keeping your upper body raised as before, and your hands palms-up on the floor. **Exhale**, stretch the front of your body to balance on your navel.

•*Take 5 deep ujjayi breaths.*

3 **Inhale**, clasp your arms behind your back and push them away from you. **Exhale**, continue to lift your chest and breathe into your heart space. Do not allow your lower back to strain in any way. Direct your gaze downward if looking forward strains your neck.

•*Take 5 deep ujjayi breaths. Then…*

FLOW OUT

Release the posture, lift your body into Four-limbed Staff (see far left), and flow into the Half Vinyasa sequence (see left and pages 64–65). End by moving from Downward Dog into an upright kneeling position.

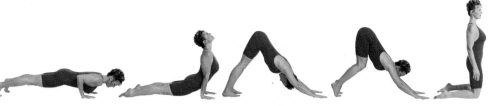

The Camel

This stress-relieving posture—*Ustrasana*—taken from the second series in the traditional *astanga vinyasa* practice (see page 6), creates a deep but safe stretch throughout your body. It is particularly useful to relieve any stiffness in the shoulders, back, and ankles of people who spend their working days sitting at desks. *Ustrasana* stretches the front of your hips, thighs, abdomen, rib cage, and throat, massages your internal organs, alleviates stomach pain, and tones your back muscles, which benefits your posture.

A Steady Gaze

As you lean back, practice *ekagra* by directing your gaze at the tip of your nose in order to soften your brow.

Only drop your head back this far if it does not strain your neck in any way. Otherwise, do the Confidence Builder (see right) instead.

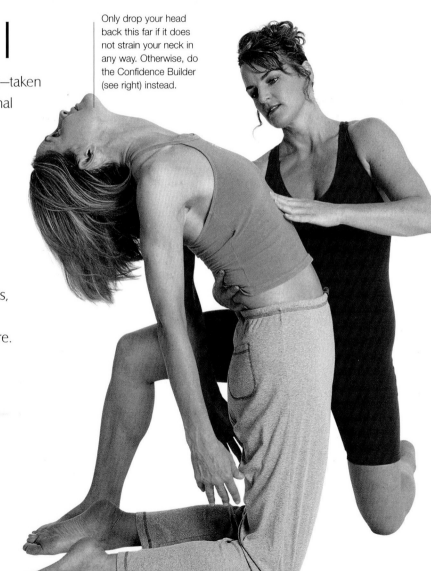

CONFIDENCE BUILDER

If this posture is too intense at first, use a stool with a pillow or folded towel on top as a support. Kneel with your back to the stool and gently lean back over the bolster so that your upper back is comfortably supported in an arch. Raise your arms above your head as you do so. Relax into the pose for up to 20 breaths if comfortable. Then rest in Child's pose (see page 7).

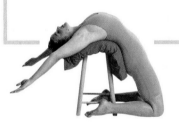

As you start to bend backward into The Camel, try to broaden across your collarbones and draw back your shoulders to help open the "back door to your heart"—your thoracic spine.

FLOW IN

Begin this pose by kneeling, with your knees hip-width apart, hips raised, toes pointed, hands by your sides, and chest lifted.

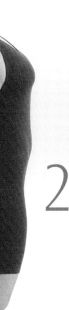

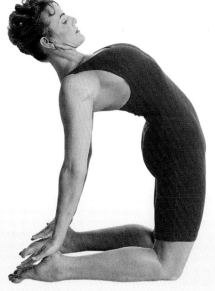

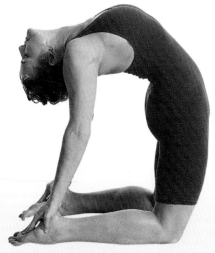

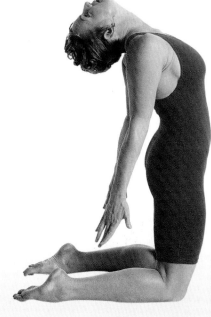

1 **Exhale**, draw your shoulders back, and place your hands on your lower back. **Inhale**, look upward.

2 **Exhale**, lift your chest upward and lean back using your thigh muscles, keeping the tops of your feet broad on the floor. **Inhale**, gradually lean further into the posture, and place your hands on your heels if you can.

•*Take 5 deep ujjayi breaths.*

3 If you are comfortable, **exhale**, lean back further to create a smooth bow in your spine by lifting your chest and drawing your shoulder blades together. Be sure to soften the back of your neck and relax your face. **Inhale**, allow your head to drop gently backward, and your hands to slide down the soles of your feet.

•*Take 5 deep ujjayi breaths.*

4 **Exhale**, ease your palms off your feet, and use the strength in your thighs to bring yourself back to upright kneeling position. **Inhale**, lift your chest and tuck your chin toward your chest as you come up to protect your neck. **Exhale**, bring your arms by your sides and look forward in an upright kneeling position. Then...

FLOW OUT

Place your hands on the floor in front of you and step back into Four-limbed Staff (see far left) to flow into the Half Vinyasa sequence (see left and pages 64–65). End by springing or stepping through from Downward Dog to Seated Staff.

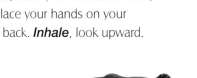
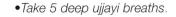

Marichyasana

Seated Twist

Twists are indispensable postures for detoxifying your body and regenerating lost energy. Named after the sage Marichi, one of the sons of the Hindu god Brahma, this lateral seated twist—*Marichyasana*—frees your spine, alleviating any pains in your back, hips, or shoulders. Also a deep stretch for your legs and torso, it massages your liver and kidneys, and removes sluggishness in your intestines. Regular practice of this pose helps to tone your waistline and your hips, and strengthen your shoulders. Make sure that you keep your back as straight as possible throughout the movement.

The Power of Visualization

Imagine that your spine is a corkscrew—turning from the base of your spine through to the base of your skull. Feel it lengthen as it twists.

CONFIDENCE BUILDER

To achieve a straight spine, practice this posture sitting on a yoga block to raise your pelvis slightly off the floor. This prevents your spine from slumping, promoting a safer, more effective rotation.

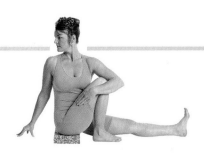

Turn the shoulder of your straight arm away and pull in your bent knee tightly. Try not to use your arms to twist you; instead, initiate the movement from your spine, turning from the core of your body.

Your fingers should be pointing away from you, and your arm should be straight but not rigid.

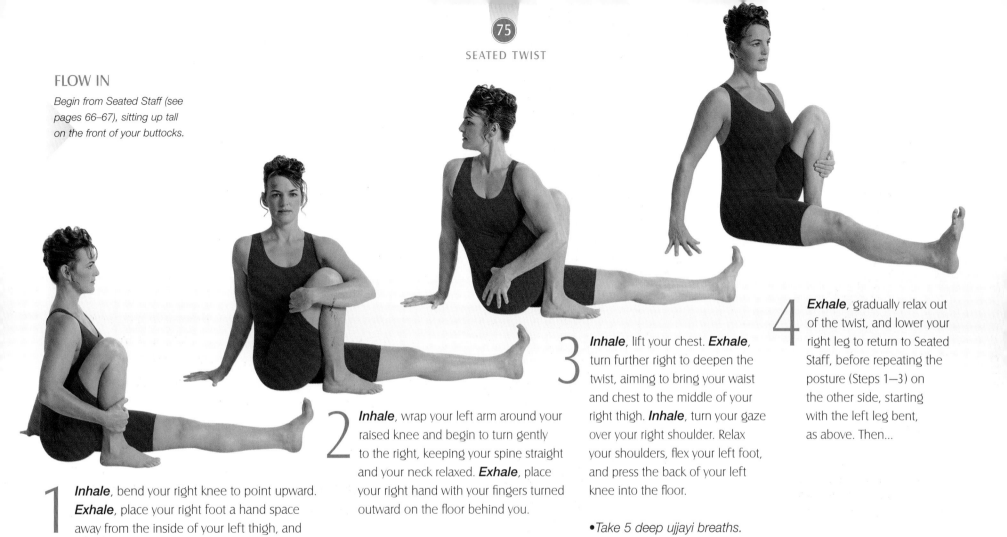

FLOW IN

Begin from Seated Staff (see pages 66–67), sitting up tall on the front of your buttocks.

1 **Inhale**, bend your right knee to point upward. **Exhale**, place your right foot a hand space away from the inside of your left thigh, and as close as possible to your right buttock.

2 **Inhale**, wrap your left arm around your raised knee and begin to turn gently to the right, keeping your spine straight and your neck relaxed. **Exhale**, place your right hand with your fingers turned outward on the floor behind you.

3 **Inhale**, lift your chest. **Exhale**, turn further right to deepen the twist, aiming to bring your waist and chest to the middle of your right thigh. **Inhale**, turn your gaze over your right shoulder. Relax your shoulders, flex your left foot, and press the back of your left knee into the floor.

•*Take 5 deep ujjayi breaths.*

4 **Exhale**, gradually relax out of the twist, and lower your right leg to return to Seated Staff, before repeating the posture (Steps 1—3) on the other side, starting with the left leg bent, as above. Then...

FLOW OUT

Return to Seated Staff. Then cross your legs to flow into the Half Vinyasa sequence (see left and pages 64–65). End by springing or stepping through from Downward Dog to Seated Staff.

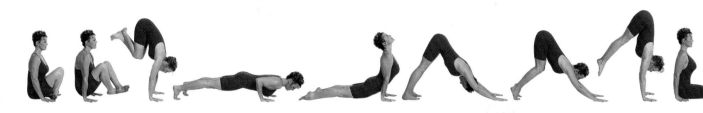

The Boat

This pose is so named because the body resembles a boat, with your arms as the oars, when in full posture. A dynamic and energizing *asana*, it considerably tones and strengthens your abdomen, back, and chest, as well as massaging your intestines. It is essential to engage *uddiyana bandha* (see page 10) in this posture to avoid straining your back. It could also be known as the Medicine pose, because it is extremely good for you, although you may not know it or like it at first due to its very challenging nature.

Mindful Breathing

Direct each deep breath into your heart and lungs to "fuel" this challenging posture.

CONFIDENCE BUILDER

If the full posture is too much, try strengthening your back by practicing the same posture but with your knees bent, and your hands cupping the backs of your upper legs, in "Half-boat."

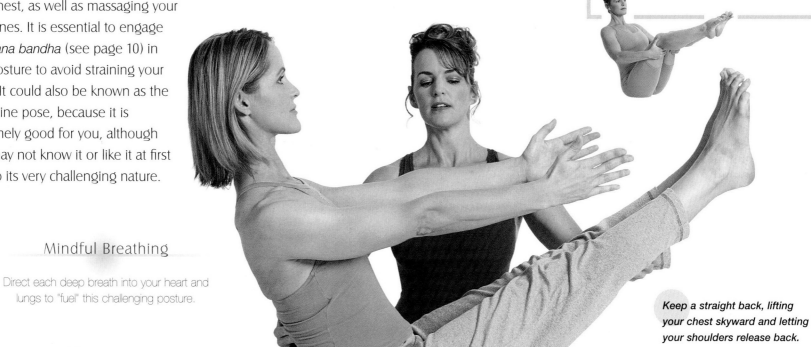

Keep a straight back, lifting your chest skyward and letting your shoulders release back.

FLOW IN

Begin from Seated Staff (see pages 66–67), making sure that you are sitting toward the front of your buttocks.

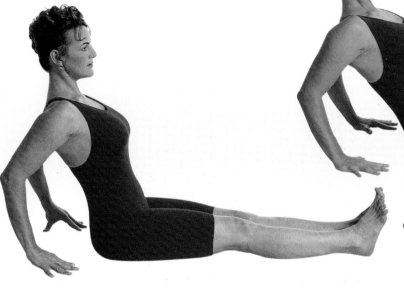

1 *Exhale*, place your hands behind you with your fingers facing forward, and lean back to create a diagonal line with your spine. *Inhale*, keep lifting your chest, and be sure to engage *uddiyana bandha* (see page 10).

2 *Exhale*, bend your arms slightly, and raise your legs diagonally up in front of you. Lift your chest, straighten your back, and create a "v" shape with your body. Make sure that you balance equally through both buttocks and keep your hands on the floor for stability.

3 If you are comfortable, *inhale*, extend your arms straight out in front of you, with your fingers pointing toward your feet. Point your toes, face your palms toward each other, and gaze forward, toward your toes. Aim to draw your chest upward with every inhalation.

•*Take 5 deep ujjayi breaths. Then…*

FLOW OUT

Return to Seated Staff. Then cross your legs to flow into the Half Vinyasa sequence (see left and pages 64–65). End by springing or stepping through from Downward Dog to Seated Staff.

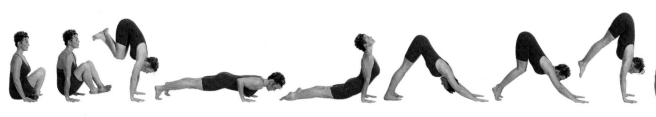

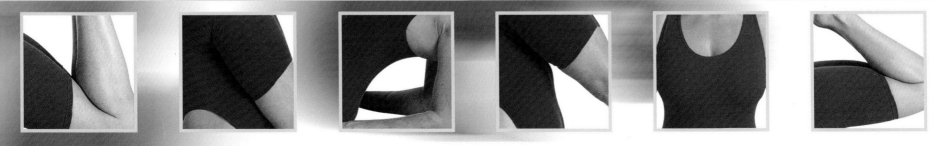

> "Cease all activity, abandon all desire; let thoughts rise and fall as they will, like the ocean's waves."

From Song of Mahamudra by Tilopa, an ancient Buddhist practitioner

The finishing postures offer your body a valuable chance to cool down and relax at the end of your dynamic yoga practice, so please do not rush them. They are just as important as all the other postures in the book, and more so if you are feeling tired.

The inverted postures (pages 80–87) replenish your mind and body, restoring depleted enegy by refreshing your internal organs and brain with vital, oxygenated blood. In fact, such is the significance of the Shoulderstand and Headstand in yoga that they are often called the queen and king of the *asanas*.

The Yogic Seal smooths the transition from finishing postures to relaxation practice. And the two relaxation practices at the end allow you to focus on breathing, meditation, and mind-cleansing—firstly in a cross-legged sitting position, and then in a supine position. Enjoy this time dedicated solely to yourself.

If the sequence becomes too challenging: rest momentarily by adopting the Child pose. This involves kneeling, sitting on your heels, bending forward to touch your head to the floor, and relaxing your arms by your sides until you feel restored and ready to continue.

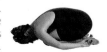

Salamba Sarvangasana

Shoulderstand

All upside-down poses are replenishing: they ease congestion in your internal organs and drain your legs of venous blood, helping to prevent varicose veins. The Sanskrit name for this, the first of the inversions—*Sarvangasana*—means "all parts posture," indicating that it cleanses and rejuvenates your entire system with yogic energy (*prana*). It brings about vitality and invigoration, coupled with calmness and repose, by allowing oxygenated blood to flow to your brain, neck, and chest. Often described as the queen of all *asanas*, it also can help to ease any breathing problems, treat colds by draining the sinuses, and clear the bowels. Anyone with specific ear, sinus, heart, or blood pressure problems, and women in the first two days of their menstrual cycle should not practice the full posture, but instead lie with their legs raised against a wall or on a chair.

The Power of Visualization

Imagine that a jug of warm liquid is being poured gently across your brow, smoothing away any tensions, and softening your face and jaw during the posture.

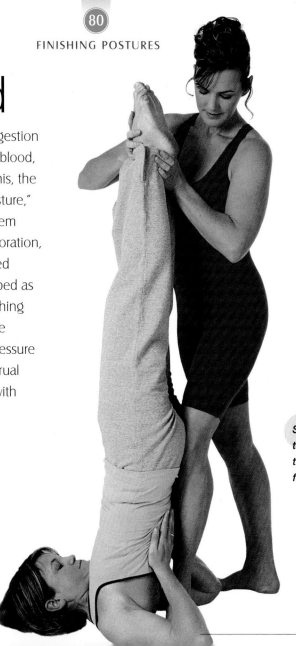

CONFIDENCE BUILDER

If the full posture is too much at first, place your palms firmly beneath the upper part of your buttocks to support your torso at a 45-degree angle, with your elbows on the floor for support. Then, straighten your legs, and bring them to an angle of 45 degrees over your body.

Stretch upward through to the tips of your toes, and try to create a straight line through your body, moving your pelvis forward to balance over your shoulders.

Make sure that you align your elbows with your shoulders so that you have a steady platform for support. And be careful not to strain your neck or move your head.

FLOW IN

Lie on your back in *Savasana*, with your legs pressed together and your toes pointed. Your head should fall slightly lower than your shoulders, so use a folded towel for support if necessary.

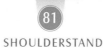

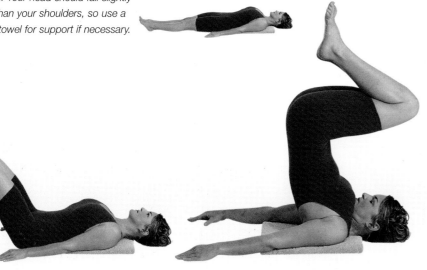

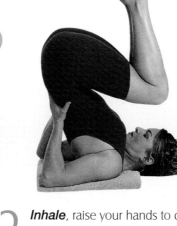

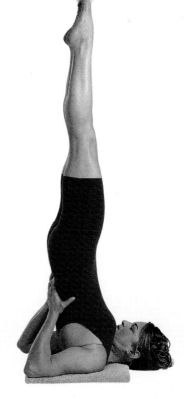

1 **Inhale**, bend your knees in toward your body, placing your feet on the floor, hip-width apart and toes facing forward. **Exhale**, tuck your chin toward your chest, and draw back your shoulders.

2 **Inhale**, press your hands down into the floor, and slowly start to lift your legs off the floor, keeping them bent at this stage. **Exhale**, press the backs of your shoulders firmly into the mat, and keep your chin tucked in. Do not move your head to either side in this pose.

3 **Inhale**, raise your hands to cup your back, and gently lower your bent knees toward your brow. Try to keep your elbows in line with your shoulders to create a square, steady platform for the posture, and to expand your chest. **Exhale**, make sure that you harness *uddiyana bandha* for abdominal support.

4 **Inhale**, straighten your legs in the air, bringing your torso and buttocks in a straight line perpendicular to the floor. **Exhale**, aim for your chest and chin to touch each other.

•*Take 20 deep ujjayi breaths. Then…*

FLOW OUT

Exhale, slowly release from the posture by bending your knees toward your forehead again, ready to flow directly into Plough.

Halasana–Karnapidasana

Plough to Ear Pressure Posture

The soothing benefits of the Shoulderstand (see pages 80–81) are enhanced in these two postures. The Plough (Steps 1–2) generally alleviates any tiredness and cools down your brain. The clasped hand position stretches your neck and opens your shoulders further, while the bend that you create in your body offers you a deep spinal stretch and massages your stomach. Flowing on from the Plough, the Ear Pressure posture (Step 3) continues this stretch of your spine and massage of your stomach, while also rejuvenating your torso, heart, and legs with healthy blood. Women in the first two days of their menstrual cycle should lie on their back and raise their legs against a wall, instead of practicing either of these two full poses.

The Power of Visualization

Relax deeply into the posture, and visualize yourself as a flower closing its petals in on itself. However, still keep the spine alert.

CONFIDENCE BUILDER

If either of these full postures are too difficult at first, bend your knees toward your forehead, with your hands cupping your back, and your elbows on the floor for support.

Concentrate on lifting your spine completely vertically, so that you keep a healthy space between your hips and your rib cage.

You can either try to place the tips of your toes on the floor or you can explore the stretch by pointing your toes away from you.

FLOW IN

Begin from having your knees bent down toward your forehead.

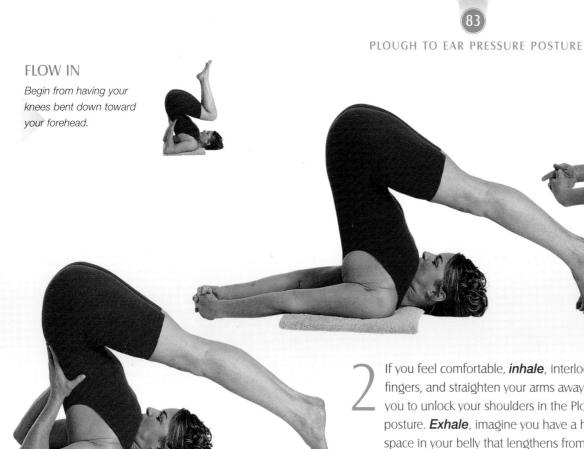

1 **Exhale**, keep your hands on your lower back for support, and straighten your legs overhead so that the tips of your toes touch the floor. Keep your hips lifted skyward and your spine as vertical as possible.

•*Take 10 deep ujjayi breaths.*

2 If you feel comfortable, **inhale**, interlock your fingers, and straighten your arms away from you to unlock your shoulders in the Plough posture. **Exhale**, imagine you have a hollow space in your belly that lengthens from your pelvis to your chest. This will drain your intestines, lengthen your lower spine, and help you maintain good posture.

•*Take 10 deep ujjayi breaths.*

3 **Inhale**, bend your knees toward your ears, aiming your lower legs toward the floor beyond your head. **Exhale**, hug your knees to your ears like headphones to seal off your hearing and encourage *pratyahara*—an inward turning, or withdrawal, of your senses. This is Ear Pressure posture and also can be practiced with your hands cupping your back as in Step 1 if you need more support.

•*Take 10 deep ujjayi breaths. Then…*

FLOW OUT

Exhale, release your hands, and gently ease your spine down into the mat. Pause to hug your legs into your abdomen, before returning to Savasana (lying flat on your back). Take one full breath, ready for Fish posture.

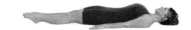

Matsyasana

The Fish

In this posture, you expand your breath into the sides of your rib cage, opening and closing them like fish gills, expanding your chest and opening your heart area. The Sanskrit texts explain that this pose enhances your ability to float in water like a fish, by moving the gravitational center to the middle of your body. The posture tones your pelvis, stretches your stomach, and is the ideal counterstretch to the three previous inverted postures. Be careful not to strain your neck when releasing your head back in this posture. Practice the Confidence Builder (see right) or stay in Step 2 (see below) if you experience any discomfort.

Mindful Breathing

Direct your breath into the bottom corners of your lungs, as if you are breathing away any "cobwebs" there.

Focus on opening the "back door to the heart"—the thoracic spine— between your shoulder blades. This should arch your upper body and lift your chest higher with every inhalation.

CONFIDENCE BUILDER

If the full posture is too hard at first, simply lean on your elbows, and lift your chest as high as you can instead. Keep your chin pressed toward your chest, and continuously draw back your shoulders.

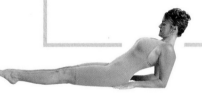

Be careful not to strain your neck as you lean your head back. Only stretch it as far as is comfortable for you.

FLOW IN

Begin from Savasana
(lying flat on your back).

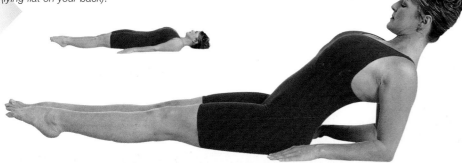

3 **Inhale**, ease your elbows down toward your hips, and remove your weight from your elbows by placing the crown of your head on the floor. If this is too intense or compresses your neck too much, remain in Step 2.

•*Take 10 deep ujjayi breaths.*

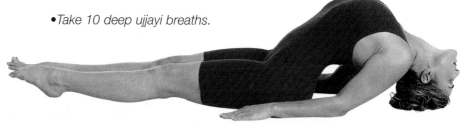

1 **Inhale**, lift up your upper body, position your elbows beneath your shoulders, and lean on them, keeping your pelvis on the floor. **Exhale**, begin to raise your chest as high as you can, with your chin tilted toward your chest and your stomach sucked in. Notice how your abdominal "suction" supports your lower back.

4 **Exhale**, gently release your head, drawing your chin toward your chest again, and keeping your elbows on the floor. **Inhale**, slowly lie down, and curl your knees into your abdomen, hugging them with your arms to provide a stretch. Ease out your lower spine by gently rocking from side to side.

•*Take 10 deep ujjayi breaths. Then…*

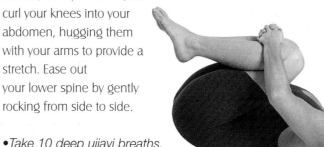

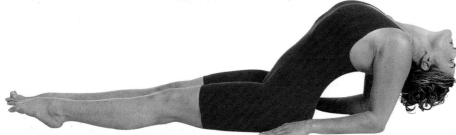

2 **Inhale**, lift your chin up, continue to lift your chest, and draw up energy through your legs, pointing your toes. **Exhale**, gently release your head back as far as is comfortable for you, broadening your collarbones.

•*Take 10 deep ujjayi breaths.*

FLOW OUT

Exhale, *roll up to sit cross-legged, before folding your mat in two to create padding for your head in the next posture. Then return to the Child pose (see left & page 7).* **Take 10 full breaths**, *ready for Headstand.*

Salamba Sirsasana

Headstand

Often referred to as king of all *asanas*, the Headstand refreshes your brain with oxygenated blood, gives your heart, and indeed all your inner organs, a rest, and allows venous blood to flow back easily to your heart, thereby cleansing your legs. This advanced posture strengthens your lungs and enriches your blood supply. Its challenging nature helps you to build stamina and enhances your ability to be fully present in the moment. It also eases any problems with your sinuses, and stimulates good digestion. Only attempt this pose once you are very confident in your yoga practice. It is highly advisable to start off by doing it with a wall behind you and/or a teacher's assistance, to avoid falling. This posture, like all inversions, should not be carried out by women during the first two days of their menstrual cycle. Do the Confidence Builder (see right) instead, or lie down on your back and raise your legs against a wall or onto a chair.

The Power of Visualization

Imagine you are a tree: your head has roots growing into the earth, through which you absorb nutrients to enrich your brain, and your feet are the branches being pulled skyward.

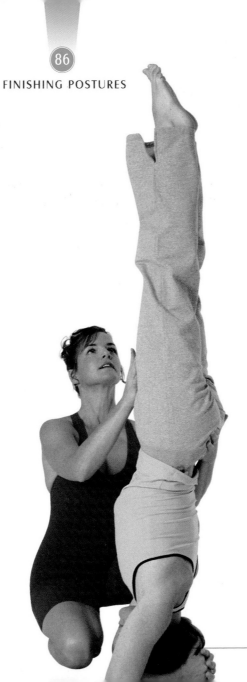

CONFIDENCE BUILDER

Alternatively, carry out Steps 1–2 below, and then clasp your hands behind your back, to gain similar benefits to those gained from Headstand. Make sure you raise your hips up, and draw your arms straight overhead in this "Raised Child" pose.

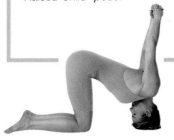

Extend yourself upward through the core of your body, pointing your toes to the sky. Make sure that you keep your tailbone tucked under and uddiyana bandha *(see page 10)* harnessed in your belly.

Only 15 percent of your weight should be on your head. Distribute the rest of your weight equally throughout the base you

FLOW IN

Begin from the Child's pose (see page 7), but raise your head and fold your elbows in front of you on your folded mat, with each hand loosely holding the opposite elbow.

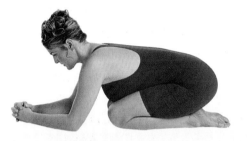

1 **Exhale**, bring your hands forward to meet each other, without moving your elbows. **Inhale**, interlock your fingers to create a cup with your hands.

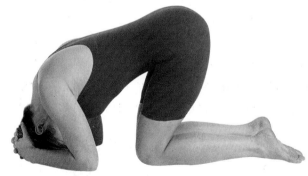

2 **Exhale**, place the top of your head onto the floor and nestle your cupped hands around the back of your head.

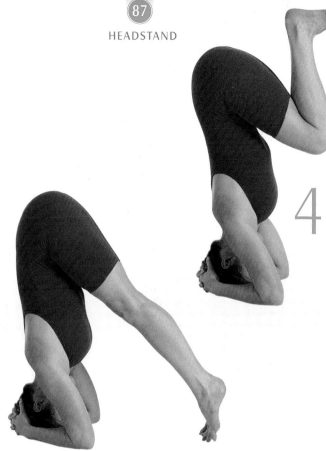

3 **Inhale**, lift your knees off the floor and tiptoe your feet toward your torso. **Exhale**, raise your hips directly above your shoulders and straighten your back. Try lifting one foot off the floor at a time to make sure that you are balanced enough for the next step. If you do not feel steady enough, remain in this position. If you do, continue with the next steps.

4 **Inhale**, lift your legs up off the floor and hug your knees into your torso. **Exhale**, keep your spine straight with the help of your *bandhas* (see page 10).

5 If you are confident and steady in this position, **inhale**, and gradually straighten your legs, balancing your pelvis above your shoulders, lengthening your spine, and lifting your shoulders away from your ears.

•*Take 20 deep ujjayi breaths. Then…*

FLOW OUT

Exhale, gently bend your knees into your torso, smoothly unfold your legs down to the floor, and return to the Child's pose. **Take 20 deep ujjayi breaths**. *Then return to Seated Staff, ready for Yogic Seal.*

Yoga Mudrasana

Yogic Seal

This pose is known as a *mudra* (yogic gesture), as it affects the mind on a deeper, more subtle level than an *asana* (posture). A *mudra* is a gesture carried out with your hands, or alternatively your feet, eyes, breath, or whole body. This *mudra*, the Yogic Seal, is ideally placed after the *asana* practice and before relaxation, as it is a gateway to deeper surrender of the mind. The pose signifies withdrawal of the senses (*pratyahara*), thus allowing you to turn your mind inward and "seal" in your energy, possibly gaining access to deeper states of consciousness. It helps to create good postural integration, to stimulate your spine, to relax your neck, and to massage your inner organs, particularly your intestines. You should experience a real sense of grounding through your pelvis when in this soothing, bent over position.

Mindful Breathing

As you bend forward, direct your breath into the backs of your lungs, and feel them filling to the brim, like bottles.

Aim to push your clasped hands away from yourself in order to open your chest and expand the space around your heart.

CONFIDENCE BUILDER

If the full posture is too intense, try folding your elbows behind your back, rather then interlocking the fingers of your straight arms. Then bend forward as in Step 3.

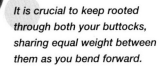

It is crucial to keep rooted through both your buttocks, sharing equal weight between them as you bend forward.

FLOW IN

Begin from Seated Staff (see pages 66–67).

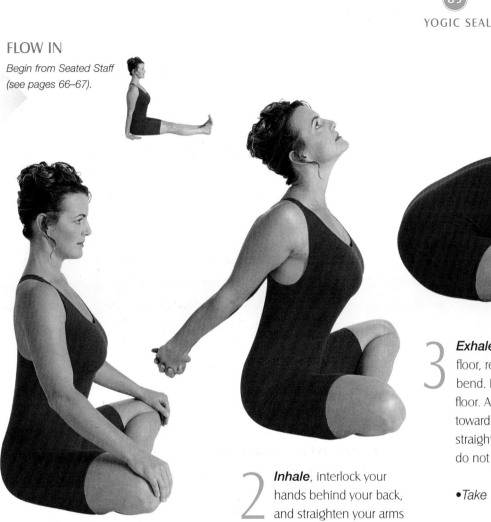

1 **Inhale**, sit in a simple cross-legged posture, *Sukhasana*. **Exhale**, lengthen your spine, and lift your chest.

2 **Inhale**, interlock your hands behind your back, and straighten your arms behind you. Then look up, keeping your brow relaxed.

3 **Exhale**, move your head toward the floor, releasing your spine into a forward bend. Keep both buttocks firmly on the floor. As you hollow your abdomen toward your spine, slowly raise your straightened arms. Don't worry if you do not get very far forward.

•*Take 10 deep ujjayi breaths.*

4 **Inhale**, gently come up and return to the cross-legged position again. **Exhale**, place your palms on the floor behind you, with your fingers spread and pointing toward your hips. **Inhale**, arch your spine, lift your chest, gently drop back your head, and broaden your collarbones.

•*Take 10 deep ujjayi breaths. Then…*

FLOW OUT

Exhale, return to the cross-legged position with your spine straight, lower your gaze, and lightly place your hands on your knees. Take 25 full breaths, ready to close your practice with Relaxation.

Seated Relaxation

Relaxation is an integral element of yoga practice, which allows your mind to slow down and escape from its usual, relentless activity. Incorporating a relaxation practice like this into your daily routine helps cultivate your powers of perception as you turn your mind inward, encouraging feelings of fragmentation to dissipate. The Seated Meditation called *metta*, meaning loving kindness, helps you relax by removing negative emotions, and cultivating *bodhicitta*, pure feelings in your heart. The practice is founded in the awareness that by being caring toward yourself first, you can then extend compassion toward others. Many emotions may arise during meditation, but the challenge is to remain still and relaxed, letting your thoughts pass on by. The *Buddha mudra* is a subtle hand gesture that helps fine-tune your mind and encourages you to relax by connecting you not only to your inner self, but also on a deeper level to the world around you.

The Power of Visualization

Strive for relaxed, compassionate focus, so that you feel as if arrows would turn to flowers if shot at your heart, as they did for Buddha when he meditated under the boddhi tree, according to Buddhist texts.

RELAXING THOUGHTS

We are what we think.
All that we are arises with our thoughts.
How can a troubled mind understand the way?
With our thoughts we make the world.
Speak or act with a pure mind
And happiness will follow you…

As spoken by Buddha in Dhammapada

Maintain the calm, seated posture with conviction and loving kindness when practicing either seated breathing metta or Buddha mudra. Stay firmly rooted through both buttocks, relax your shoulders, and keep your spine straight.

Find a place away from distraction, such as a dimly lit room where artificial stimulus is minimal. Sit cross-legged on the floor, close your eyes, quieten your mind as much as possible, and begin to observe your breath internally.

METTA: LOVING KINDNESS

Gently rest your hands, palms-up, on your knees. Breathe deeply, letting your thoughts float by like clouds through the sky. Visualize yourself bathed in soft white light that makes you feel positive and loving. Then imagine a friend of yours beside you, also surrounded by this comforting light. Next, create this loving visualization for an acquaintance, and finally do it for someone who you do not like so much. This will cleanse you of negative thoughts and develop your sense of compassion and contentedness. Remain cross-legged with your spine straight, your eyes closed, and your hands, palms-up, on your knees.

You may wish to add *Buddha mudra* to your Seated Relaxation practice—the hand gesture that Buddha is said to have adopted during his quest for enlightenment under the boddhi tree.

BUDDHA MUDRA

Sitting cross-legged, point your left hand downward so that your fingers touch the floor in front of your left knee, signifying your deep connection to the earth. Leave your right hand on your right knee, but touch your index finger and thumb together to form a circle, signifying your connection on a deeper level with the world around you. These hand gestures symbolize the importance of fulfilling earthly obligations, while also being able to see beyond the mundane, physical world to a more enlightened, spiritual way of living.

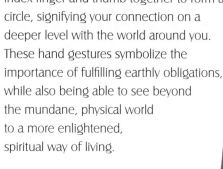

The position of this hand is known as *jnana mudra* and the touch of your thumb and fingertip symbolizes the union of individual consciousness with universal consciousness.

Final Relaxation

Adopting the "corpse" posture—*Savasana*—gives you the chance to remove yourself from all activity by lying completely still. While relaxing on your back, your parasympathetic nervous system takes over, giving your overused sympathetic nervous system a well-deserved break from the excitement, anxiety, and stress that often send it into overdrive. This eases your nerves, lifts any feelings of anxiety or depression, lets you focus on effortless breathing, and gives your body some much-needed recovery time to restore its balance and harmony. This is particularly important after this vigorous yoga program. Bear in mind that deep relaxation should mean alert, but relaxed, attention, not a dull sleep. Remain fully aware and observe how your body feels after its mental and physical yoga practice. Breathe deeply throughout.

The Power of Visualization

To help you relax, imagine a tiny golden star in the center of your brain. Watch it grow until its golden light surrounds you, making you feel secure. Then watch it gradually melt away again, allowing you to rest with a clear mind.

RELAXING THOUGHTS

Do naught with the body but relax, Shut firm the mouth and silent remain, Empty your mind and think of naught. Like a hollow bamboo, rest at ease with your body. Giving not, nor taking, put your mind at rest.

From Song of Mahamudra, by Tilopa

Ease your spine gently into the floor, vertebra by vertebra, from your lower spine right through to your shoulders, the nape of your neck, and your head.

KEEP WARM

Cover yourself with a blanket or put on a sweatshirt if you start to feel cold at any point.

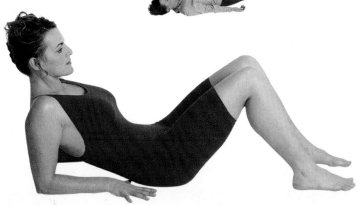

1 **Inhale**, sit with your knees bent and pointing up, and your feet parallel on the floor. **Exhale**, lean back onto your elbows.

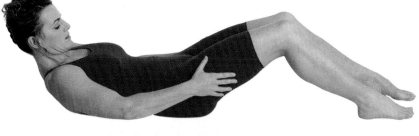

2 Breathing deeply, gradually uncurl your spine into the floor. Enjoy the feeling of weight as your muscles relax into the floor.

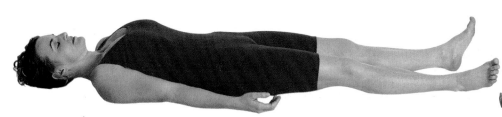

3 Let both sides of your body relax into the floor, allowing your arms and legs to rest, with your palms facing upward and your toes falling outward. Then close your eyes, relax your jaw, and let your shoulders become heavy. Focus on your breathing, letting your abdomen rise as you inhale, and fall as you exhale.

• *Rest here for at least 10 minutes.*

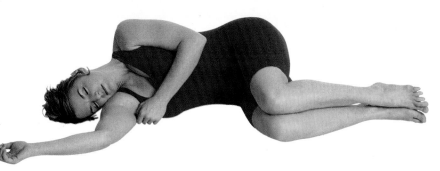

4 Slowly begin to move your fingers and toes, your hands and feet, your arms and legs, and then your head. Once fully stretched, roll over to rest on your right side, until you are ready to end your yoga practice by returning to a seated position.

Glossary

Abdomen the stomach area

Ahimsa Buddhist term meaning non-violence

Asana posture, meaning to "sit in steadiness"

Bandha a subtle, internal lock used to seal energy within your body during yoga practice

Bodhicitta Buddhist term for pure feelings, heart essence, or positive emotional energy

Cervical spine uppermost part of your spine, consisting of seven vertebrae in your neck

"Charge" mobilize, engage, or activate muscular support around your joints and bones

Collarbones bones in your upper chest that join your breastbone and shoulder blades

Colon part of your large intestine

"Core of the body" the center of gravity for your body, based where your pelvis and spine meet

Drishti gaze point

Ekagra a single focus for your gaze, which helps bring your mind to a still point

Endocrine system the internal system that controls many basic human functions through the secretion of hormones by glands

"Energetic lightness" a lack of internal sluggishness and lack of heaviness in your body

"Firm foundation" core stability in your postures

Heartspace term for the area around your heart

Jalandhara bandha throat lock used to seal energy within your body during yoga practice

Kundalini latent energy in your body, often symbolized by a coiled serpent

Lumbar spine lower region of your back, consisting of five vertebrae between your ribs and your pelvis

Mantra sacred sound—usually a meaningful phrase repeated for a specific effect

Metta Buddhist term for "loving kindness"

Mudra symbolic hand gesture

Mula bandha lock at the base of your pelvis, used to seal energy within your body during yoga practice

Muscle organ specialized for contraction to produce body movement

Nadis subtle nerves in yogic energy, akin to meridian channels in Chinese acupuncture

Namaste Sanskrit term for a yogic hand position, also known as "prayer position"

Organ structure composed of two or more different tissues with a specific, vital function

Parasympathetic nervous system the part of the nervous system that conserves and restores energy

Pelvic basin bone structure at your pelvis, where your hip bones, sacrum, and coccyx meet

Perineum fibrous nodule in your pelvic floor between your anus and genitals

Prana yogic term for vital energy or life force

Pranayama breath control used in yoga

Pratyahara conscious withdrawal of your senses

Primary series initial sequence of *astanga vinyasa* yoga postures, as taught by Sri K. Patthabi Jois in Mysore, India, to align your body and mind

Samskara the cycle of being caught up in conditioned reactions or habitual tendencies

Second series intermediate group of postures in *astanga vinyasa* yoga, to be practiced after the primary series in order to cleanse your system

Shoulder blades the large, flat bones of your upper back

Sinus hollow area in a bone or other tissue that acts as a channel for your blood

"Sitting bones" the bones in your bottom, upon which you sit

Spine backbone, consisting of seven cervical, twelve thoracic, and five lumbar vertebrae from your skull to the small of your back

Sternum breastbone at the center of your chest

Sympathetic nervous system part of the nervous system concerned with expenditure of energy

"Third eye" yogic term for the space between your eyebrows, which relates to intuition and discernment

Thoracic spine middle part of your spine

Thorax the section of your body in which your heart and lungs are positioned

Thyroid gland gland in your throat that secretes a hormone governing your metabolism

Uddiyana bandha subtle abdominal lock used to seal energy within your body during yoga practice

***Ujjayi* breath** controlled, deep breathing technique specific to *astanga vinyasa* yoga and created by adopting the *bandhas*

Vein vessel carrying blood back to your heart

Venous blood blood returning to your heart through your veins

Vertebra each individual segment of your spine

Visceral referring to the vital organs of your body

"Wingspan" symbolic term for the area across your upper back

Acknowledgments

A HUGE THANK YOU to the expert crew at Carroll & Brown for the fun we had making this book: Jules Selmes, Justin Ford, David Yems, and especially my editor, Kelly Thompson, who has been a solid and inspiring joy to work with.

Thanks also to the yogis who modelled, adding positive energy to the project: Jenny Smith, Caroline Hilmy, Graham Stones, and Kelly Thompson.

Liz Lark

Carroll & Brown would also like to thank Jesse Owen for hair and make up; and Michelle Bernard for indexing the book.

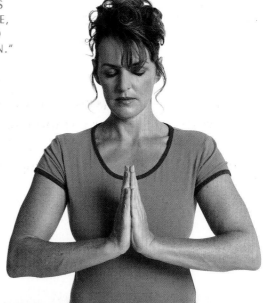

"AT FIRST THE YOGI FEELS LIKE THE MIND IS TUMBLING LIKE A WATERFALL IN MID-COURSE, LIKE THE GANGES, IT FLOWS ON SLOW AND GENTLE; IN THE END IT IS LIKE A VAST OCEAN."

FROM THE SONG OF MAHAMUDRA, BY TILOPA

Index